Thirsk

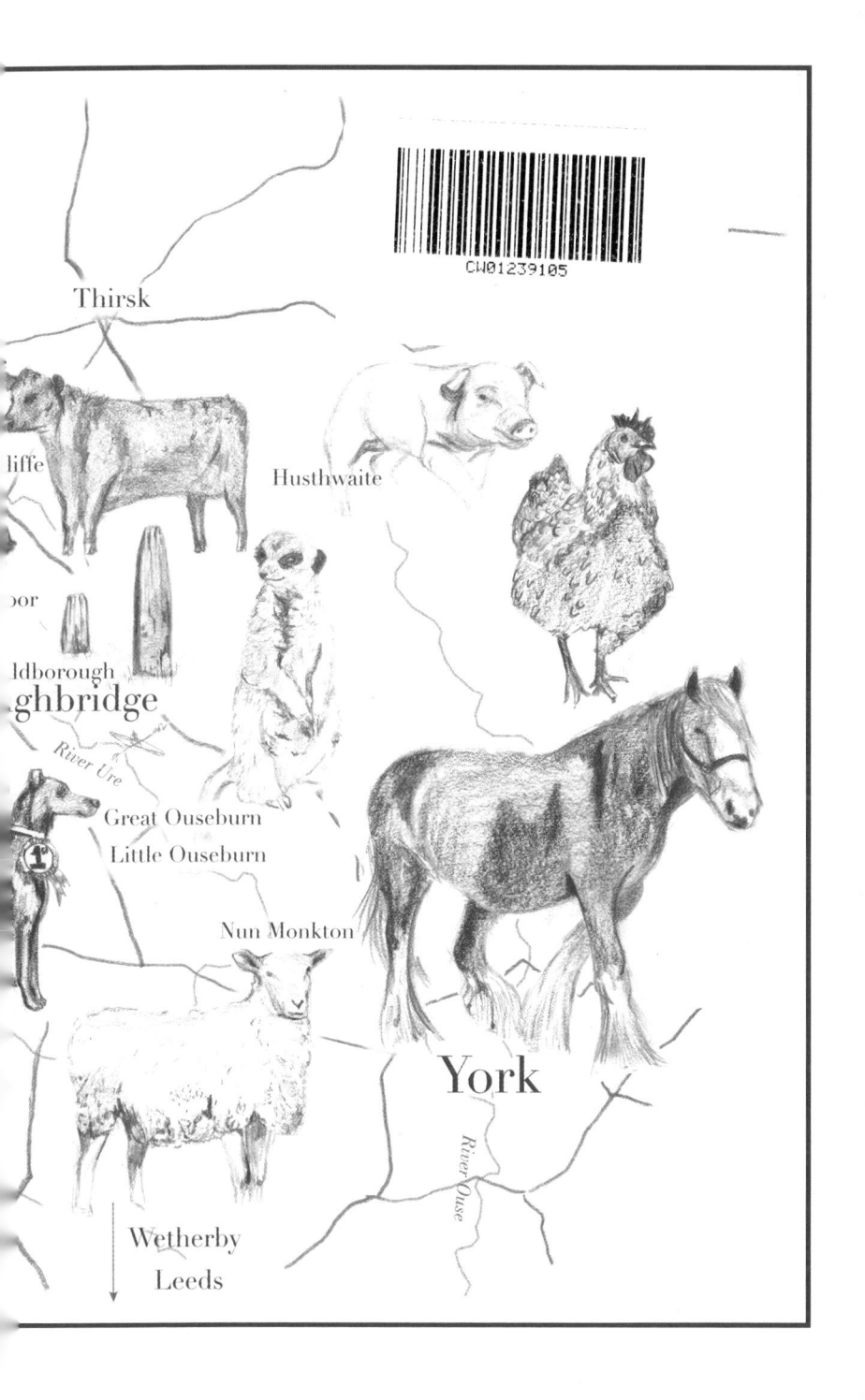

liffe

Husthwaite

oor

ldborough
ghbridge

River Ure

Great Ouseburn
Little Ouseburn

Nun Monkton

York

River Ouse

Wetherby
Leeds

a signed edition from
GREAT NORTHERN

RUMINATIONS of a YORKSHIRE VET

JULIAN NORTON

GREAT NORTHERN

Great Northern Books Limited
PO Box 1380, Bradford, BD5 5FB
www.greatnorthernbooks.co.uk

© Julian Norton 2024

Every effort has been made to acknowledge correctly and contact the copyright holders of material in this book. Great Northern Books Limited apologises for any unintentional errors or omissions, which should be notified to the publisher.

All rights reserved. No part of this book may be reproduced in any form or by any means without permission in writing from the publisher, except by a reviewer who may quote brief passages in a review.

ISBN: 978-1-914227-63-9

Design and layout: David Burrill

CIP Data
A catalogue for this book is available from the British Library

MIX
Paper | Supporting responsible forestry
FSC® C016779

Contents

Introduction 5
Springtime on the Farm 7
Udder in Whixley 9
Discretion Is the Better Part of Valais 11
It's Only Undercoat 13
Eating the Wrong Things 15
Fish on Its Side 17
Forty-Eight Hours in May 19
Hit the Hotspot 21
RTS Again 23
Princess with the Back End Injury 25
Nelly with Legs Like an Elephant 27
Cute Puppy with a Strange Eye 29
Burton Leonard 31
The Great Yorkshire Show 33
The Curious Incident of the Dog on Sunday Morning 35
This week I Have Been Mostly Sticking My Finger Up Dogs' Bums .. 38
Bull's Eye, Owl's Eye 40
Grass Seed in Eye 42
Just Chuck it up, Duck. 44
Betty 46
There's a Goose, Loose in the Lane 48
Tom's DA 51
Tom's DA Continued 53
Alpaca in the Practice. 55
Another Alpaca in the Practice. 57
Stanley and His Semen 59
Pregnant but Broken 61
Milk Fever 63
Enzo and His Bad Eye 65
Podcast 67
Confusacat 69
Goldfish, Open Mouth and Fake News 71
Tiny Tim and Painful Prostates 73
Back to Back 75

Christmas at the Vet's	77
Stories of New Year's Eve Past	79
I've Got a Fleam	82
Duck Hunt	84
Back to Work	87
Eating Onions	90
Boris and Luna	92
Two Crocks	94
Alpacas on the Telly	96
Chateauneuf du Hamster	99
Coronavirus. Or Actual Facts	102
Hedgehog Three Legs	104
Reel Around the Fountain	106
Rescued from a Spanish Ravine	108
It's You-thanasia	111
Life in a Time of Corona 1	113
Life in a Time of Corona 2	115
Life in a Time of Corona 3	117
Life in a Time of Corona 4	119
Life in a Time of Corona 5	121
Life in a Time of Corona 6	123
Spleen Out	126
New Life, Cicero and Tacitus	128
Keeping Your Head	130
Life in a Time of Corona 7	133
Prolapses Two Times and Scooby the World's Most Unlucky Cat	135
The Dog that Said 'Hello'	137
Butcher's Dog	139
Minty Gloves	142
Zoomed Out	144
Pulling Feet	146
Pigs	148
Fleeced	151
Baby Ferrets and Cria Kindergarten	153
Goat with a Hairdo	155
Vasectomising a Tup	157
The Effects of Telly	159

Introduction

Over the last eight or nine years, my professional life has been more exciting and less predictable than a typical veterinarian's. I've been involved in a returning TV series, *The Yorkshire Vet* – Channel 5's popular show, currently in its eighteenth series – and I continue to write books (this one is the ninth). I've moved jobs, to continue my passion for independent practice, which has brought huge turmoil and plenty of challenges. One of the constants, since 2016, has been my weekly missive to *The Yorkshire Post*.

The routine and discipline of thinking what to write about, penning the words, then re-reading and re-writing to knock the piece into a succinct 630 words or so has been very satisfying. The columns put forward the view and experiences of a mixed practitioner during lockdown and Covid-19 and touch on the subtle and continued shift in farming and the veterinary industry. Some of them throw a light on stories I've been part of in *The Yorkshire Vet*, always carefully treading the path between providing a glimpse without giving away the details of the story – not always easy. And I've related amusing anecdotes as accurately as I could. I've obtained permission, or used altered names, for patients and clients, to maintain professionalism and client confidentiality, usually but not always successfully! I've reminisced about past pleasures and some not so good experiences, such as the Foot and Mouth Crisis. And I've described the journey of helping to establish two new, independent practices in the county.

Some of my first *Yorkshire Post* contributions have been collated before. *The Diary of a Yorkshire Vet* and *On Call with a Yorkshire Vet* were neatly collected and published by Great Northern Books, a good old local publisher. I thought there might be people who would be interested in the short stories who didn't read *The Yorkshire Post*. These books might hopefully keep the stories alive, rather than for wrapping up fish and chips or filling the recycling bin, allowing them to diffuse beyond the boundaries of our county.

This book – the first of three – is another collection of my anecdotes that first appeared in *The Yorkshire Post* and covers some of the time I spent in the quaint and historic town of Boroughbridge. The practice where I worked during this time was just as traditional as the town and it had "Herriot" charm in abundance. It also covers the traumatic period of the outbreak of COVID-19. So, if you have picked up this book and decided to take it to the counter to buy, be warned: it is more than just a handful of animal anecdotes . . .

I hope you enjoy it!

Springtime on the Farm

Last week was a busy one for me, as it was for everyone connected with farming at this time of year. Lambing has been as hectic as ever, although, maybe as a consequence of last year's terrible spring, many farmers seem to be lambing a bit later. This spreads the work out a bit for us, which is good. Calving, too, seems to be less demanding than it often can be. Some are ascribing this to a long winter followed by a very dry summer last year – the result seems to be slightly smaller calves. Many factors are at work though, and the wrong choice of bull or a misjudgement in the feeding regime of heifers over the latter part of pregnancy can upset the best laid plans of men. And mice, although I've never had to deliver a mouse.

But the week was busy, not just because of the usual seasonal work, but because I took on the role of "Springtime Vet" on another Channel 5/Daisybeck spectacular, *Springtime on the Farm*. As I write, I can just hear Lindsey Chapman's dulcet tones as she announces the pre-titles.

Cannon Hall Farm in South Yorkshire played host to the event, which is now in its second year and rapidly becoming another Channel 5 favourite, following in and next to the footsteps of *The Yorkshire Vet*. I was delighted to be a part of this programme again. It is a very different experience to my usual telly stuff. There is a "set" or "studio", there are lights, cameras everywhere and jibs to allow swinging camera shots and interesting angles. We have to wear earpieces so we can hear feedback from the director's office, and there are autocues for the presenters (but not for the likes of me – I have to make it up as I go along!)

It's an unusual world to have landed in, but on the days I was a guest on the show, I was lucky enough to have some real veterinary work to do. On the first day, I was filmed carrying out a pregnancy scan on a heifer. She had been negative on her first scan, so had been served again by the bull. By the time I scanned her again, she should have been six weeks' pregnant – a perfect time to see a foetus and its heart beat live on the programme! Sadly, the heifer was not pregnant for a second time so there was no magic TV moment on that occasion.

The following day I had to vacate my position on the sofa, where I was supposed to be discussing modern veterinary health strategies to improve welfare, reduce disease and limit the use of antimicrobials, to attend to a ewe with ringwomb. This is a condition whereby the ewe goes into labour but the cervix fails to dilate, so the lambs cannot be born. It is often possible to open the cervix with gentle manipulation but sometimes it is necessary to perform an emergency caesarean section. Luckily, the lambs were both quite small and I was able to deliver them by the normal route.

My third day on the farm saw me back in the lambing shed, this time to replace and suture a vaginal prolapse. The pesky prolapse had been popping out repeatedly over the preceding few days, stubbornly refusing to follow Robert and David's plan of using a plastic "retainer". These spatula-shaped devices usually work well to keep a grapefruit-sized prolapse in position, but on this occasion things hadn't gone to plan. For the third time, I found myself explaining a veterinary procedure, this time with the straining back end of a sheep pointing directly to camera. I hope the editors were kind!

Udder in Whixley

Richard called me first thing on Saturday morning. He was worried about his cow. She had calved two days before and she hadn't eaten her breakfast. This is a sure sign that a cow is not well. Cows love their food, especially soon after they have had a calf, when they need as much energy as possible to provide the calf with plenty of milk. The experienced farmer knew something was wrong.

I put him down first on my long list of visits for the morning. I had a lot to do. Luckily, the patient and her calf were ready and waiting for me when I arrived and so was Richard. I climbed over the gate, into the large, straw-filled pen.

"I'm just not sure what's wrong with her," Richard explained, worried and confused in equal measure. I set about my examination as usual, asking questions as I went along about how the calving had gone, whether the cow had cleansed and so on.

"Her eyes look half closed as if she has a headache," he said, bemused.

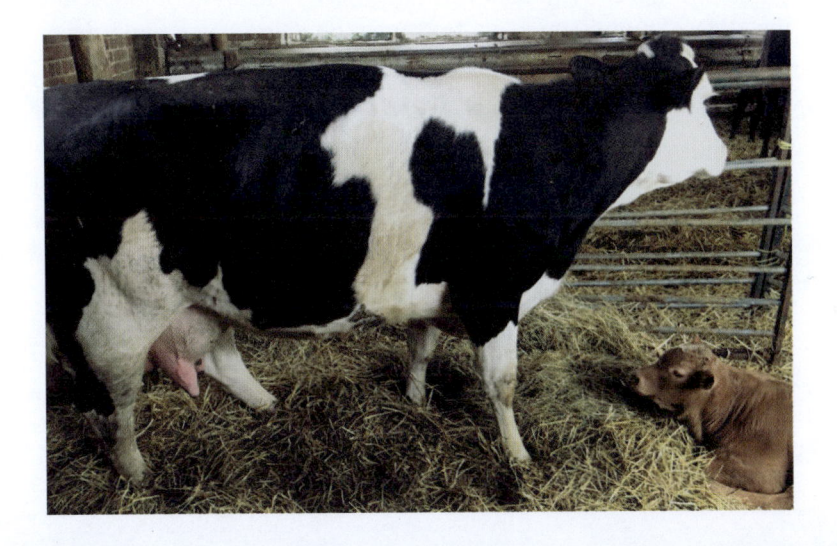

Richard was right, she did look poorly and I could imagine that she did have a splitting headache, although, of course, there was no real way of telling. The silence that met me when I listened to her rumen with my stethoscope told me she had not eaten anything for a while and when I looked at my thermometer it was clear she was very sick: her temperature was 104 degrees, which was sky-high for a cow and indicative of an infection. I checked her udder and gently pulled on each teat to check the milk. Part of her udder was pinky-red, which was a sign of possible mastitis, and as we peered at the milk that I'd extracted from each quarter, I noticed some little flecks in one of the samples. The cow had mastitis and the infection had started to spread into her system, the cause of her fever. It was definitely in the early stages – more advanced illness causes a swollen and hot udder and the milk can be brown, bloodstained and watery and can even have the fetid smell associated with an abscess. Richard was on the ball today, which was good for the cow and her chances of recovery, but harder for the vet, looking for more subtle signs of disease.

In days gone by, when cattle had vague signs of illness like this, in its early stages, before clinical signs had developed, veterinary surgeons would pronounce that the animal had a "chill". At a follow-up examination the next day, the source of the infection would have become more obvious (maybe in the udder, the lungs, the uterus, or even a swollen joint) and the vet would pronounce with confidence that "the chill has settled in the lungs/udder/knee joint" etc. But this Saturday morning, I'd managed to identify the problem. I gave my patient two injections – one of antibiotics and the other of non-steroidals – to combat infection, fever and sepsis, and said I'd come back the next day. Not to find out where the chill had settled, but to ensure she was responding to my treatment.

On Sunday morning I went back, as promised. The cow and calf were in exactly the same shed and I pulled up next to the gate and hopped over, just as I had the previous day. Whilst this bit seemed like déjà vu, the cow was different altogether. Her eyes were wide, silage was emerging from each side of her mouth and her rumen was churning over nicely. The udder was a normal, healthy flesh colour – not red or inflamed: she was on the mend and both cow and calf would soon be heading out to grass, happy and healthy.

Discretion Is the Better Part of Valais

My morning was shaping up to be busy and I had a visit to fit in before embarking on an ops list that would surely take me well into the afternoon. The biggest operation of the morning was on a rabbit called Percy. He had a bad eye. I'd seen him a couple of times over recent weeks, but the swollen globe was refusing to respond to treatment and so the decision had been made to remove it.

Coincidentally, Percy's owner was an optometrist. Once he had told me this, everything became very much easier because I could describe the pathology that I could see in the rabbit's eye in technical terms. It was red and swollen but, surprisingly, not obviously painful. I was concerned about a condition called glaucoma, where pressure builds inside the eyeball causing all sorts of problems and often blindness. There is a piece of kit called a tonometer that measures the pressure inside the eye, but it is a tool not many vets can run to, so it generally falls to specialist ophthalmologists who have this expensive equipment to test objectively for glaucoma.

But Percy was lucky – his owner had a tonometer and assured me that Percy's eyes would be tested and measured by the time he returned for a follow-up visit.

However, his owner had one concern. "How do I know what normal is, for a rabbit, I mean?" he asked.

"Well, just measure the pressure in his good eye as well as the bad one," I suggested. "That way we'll know for sure."

Lo and behold, the pressure in the bad eye was over 30mmHg (the units for measuring pressure), compared to around 12mmHg in the normal eye. This was a sure sign that Percy needed surgery. Upsetting as it can be, in a swollen, blind and unresponsive eye, surgery to remove it is the best thing and offers a simple option to alleviate the pain and solve the problem quickly.

Everything went smoothly and Percy was soon sitting up back in his kennel, looking (with just one eye) for his tasty greens to kick-start his recovery from the anaesthetic.

I left Percy to recover, as another emergency demanded my attention. This time it was a lamb and a rare one at that. It was one of Rob's last lambs to be born this springtime and was a rare breed called a Swiss Valais, which hails from the Bernese Oberland and the other high mountains of the upper reaches of the Rhone. I've been there recently on a ski tour, although I didn't see any of these amazing-looking sheep. The mountains seemed a million miles away as I worked out how best to treat this cute little lamb, with its fluffy features and black face, with a mop of frizzy white fleece on top of its head, just like a football player from the 1980s. The birth had been smooth, but the ewe had been overzealous in her attempts to clean up the lamb and had somehow trodden on the little baby and broken his front leg. The fracture was a bad one – quite high up the leg and very unstable and it would certainly need a careful repair. I opted for a modern fibreglass cast – one which is strong and light and would be perfect to facilitate a good recovery. The more old-fashioned plaster of Paris, often used for this procedure, is heavy and less supportive.

For the second time in a day, I decided that discretion was the better part of Valais.

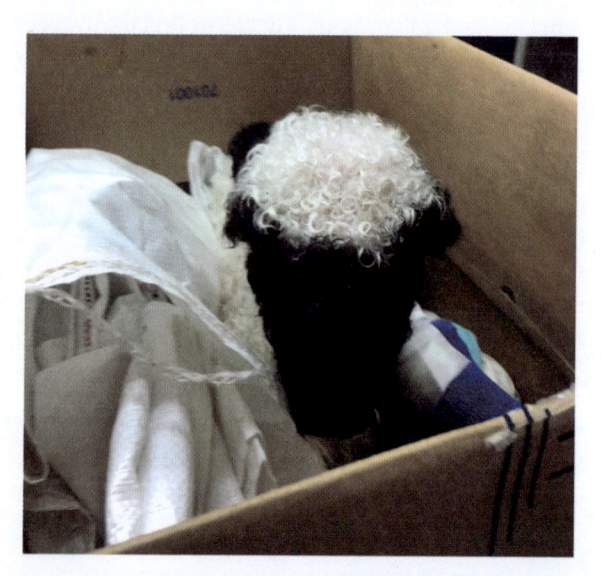

It's Only Undercoat

Saturday morning surgery was always going to be a challenge. Not only was the appointment list fully booked up before Thursday had finished, but we also had the decorators in.

Repainting the clinical areas of a veterinary practice is a nightmare. This is mainly because it has to be fitted around normal work, but also because everything has to be moved and put in boxes, out of the way of the painters and their pots. It is hard enough to find some bits of equipment even in non-decorating circumstances. Horse vets have a habit of removing essential bits of kit to take on their visits and nurses keep moving things around in their continued quest for clean-and-tidiness. It did not augur well for a relaxing morning.

Boroughbridge was looking resplendent in the late spring sunshine and the visitors were out in force, many of them calling in at the surgery to say hello or take photos of the practice from the street. At least the first layer of paint had already been applied before we opened, and it seemed to have dried. The classic charcoal matt finish of the undercoat looked quite stylish, though we all knew it was only temporary, soon to be covered up by the blue gloss that characterises the surgery.

As the patients and the visitors came and went, it seemed all was progressing smoothly. The diabetic cat I'd seen earlier in the week, suffering from laryngitis, had responded better than either the owner or I had expected. "I'm so pleased, Julian," commented her relieved owner, as she handed over a box of chocolates. "I think we all thought it was the diabetes going wrong, but to realise it was a separate condition was absolutely marvellous."

One of the last patients of the morning was a terrier called Bella, who had also been in the practice earlier in the week. She, too, was back for a check-up.

It turned out I knew Bella and her owners from a previous existence, but hadn't recognised her when she had been in earlier in the week, mainly because she had been in so much pain – yelping and crying out and trying to bite anyone who approached because of a back injury sustained falling off a wall. X-rays had not shown any serious problems, and the feisty little Patterdale had responded superbly well to treatment. My first job, after calling her and her owners through, was to apologise for not recognising them or the dog.

"Well, Julian, as you can see, she's a completely different dog now," her owners related. I examined her as best as I could – her typical Patterdale Terrier demeanour had returned and she didn't want me to fiddle with her any more than was absolutely necessary.

"She's been taking the medicine and we've been very strict with her activity, as we were told. She doesn't like the cage she's been in, but we've been keeping her very restricted," reported Mum, as she repeatedly tried to stop Bella from jumping up at the door of the consulting room.

Bella was definitely intent on leaving and, whenever she thought nobody was watching her, she was back up on her back feet, trying to get to the handle of the newly painted door.

"Stop it, Bella. Get down!" exclaimed her owner.

"It's OK – don't worry about it," I said, to save the little dog any further castigation. "It's just the undercoat. She won't do it any harm."

"I'm not bothered about your paint, Julian! It's her back I'm worried about. Your colleague said she wasn't allowed to jump up at anything!"

We all fell around laughing at the obvious, comical misunderstanding. The little dog was definitely on the mend.

Eating the Wrong Things

Dogs have an uncanny knack of eating all sorts of inappropriate things. Sometimes this can be very serious, necessitating prompt, often surgical, intervention. In other cases the consequences can be quite minor and occasionally amusing. Around Easter, there is always the problem of chocolate and foil to upset a dog's digestive system, but most of Easter's chocolate eggs have been finished off by now, and the two cases I saw this week were different again.

The first was a dog, who had eaten some rat poison whilst away with his owners, who were visiting friends. Upon returning to Yorkshire, his owners made the phone call, to alert me to the incident. Unfortunately, because the dietary indiscretion happened in Somerset, some five hours previously, there was no merit whatsoever in making the hapless canine vomit, because the poison (which, mercifully, sounded like just a few granules rather than a whole packet) would have long since passed out of the stomach and into the intestines. Rat poison causes fatal bleeding in its victims, by disrupting the pathways that lead to blood clotting when required. Luckily for the terrier, there is an excellent antidote, which I arranged to dispense to pre-empt these toxic effects.

My second case of the week did not require any specific intervention from me. Ebby the Labrador had eaten the packet of desiccant that accompanied some new clothes, which her owner had been trying on.

"My husband has some new shorts for work and this packet fell out on the floor and the dozy dog ate it immediately," explained the lady over the phone.

My immediate response was to ask what job her husband did that necessitated wearing shorts. I had just returned from probably the last lambing of the spring, in an unseasonably cold rain storm, from which I still hadn't warmed up. I couldn't imagine why anyone would be requiring shorts for work. However, this wasn't really the issue I needed to address, so I tried to move on to matters of a veterinary nature. But before I could, the lady continued,

"And then my husband made her sick and the packet came out, almost whole, but with the top bit missing. That must be still inside her."

Again, my mind wandered from the veterinary questions and I found myself following up this with the question, "How did your husband make her sick? Just out of interest, I mean."

Usually powerful emetic drugs or strong soap is required to precipitate ejection of the contents of a dog's stomach, so I was intrigued to hear what non-veterinary method had been employed.

"Well, you see, my husband has worked with pigs all his life. He's transported them all over the world. He stuck his fingers down her throat and she was sick immediately," explained the owner. One question had been answered, although I couldn't fully understand why a pig haulier would necessarily have the skills to induce vomiting in a dog.

"And what is she doing now? Is she poorly?" I asked, keen to get a fuller clinical picture.

"Well, she's certainly sheepish – she knows she's done something wrong," came the reply. "Wait a minute, I'll ask my husband." Then, after a short pause, "She's eating some gaffer tape."

There's no helping some dogs, but I felt happy that Ebby would be fine without further emetics. I issued instructions about what to look out for over the next day or so, in case the clinical picture changed. As I sat back with a cup of coffee and a veterinary magazine, the first article caught my eye. The headline read: *Miracle dog survives after eating a Nintendo DS games console.* My cases this week seemed very mundane by comparison!

Fish on Its Side

I don't get to treat many fish. This is not a bad thing, because they are not very easy to examine, diagnostic tests are limited and there are only a few treatment options available. Luckily for me, the fish I saw this week had a very obvious problem. Jeff the Fancy Goldfish (I presume named Jeff Goldfish after the American actor Jeff Goldblum) was swimming on his side. This is a classic sign of swim bladder disease.

Fancy Goldfish are, compared with other fish, not brilliant at swimming. This is partly because of their short, fat body shape and partly because of the arrangement of their fins, which are more suited to aesthetics than function – the equivalent of knee-length Bermuda shorts versus Speedos. The swim bladder is an internal structure, which aids buoyancy. In short, fat goldfish this is squashed and sometimes bent, so it doesn't work as well as it would in a more streamlined fish. It is an accident waiting to happen.

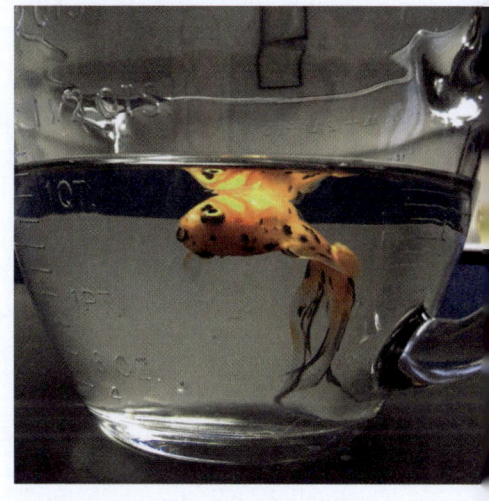

Jeff's owner lifted the tea towel off the large, glass jug in which Jeff had been transported to the surgery. The little fish was definitely very lop-sided and certainly it was his distorted and swollen swim bladder that was causing him to list.

As is usually the case, Jeff did not seem unduly distressed, although it is hard to tell if a goldfish is happy or not. I didn't need to do any diagnostic tests – the condition could be handled by management of Jeff's diet. Firstly, he was to have nothing to eat for a day, then he needed a change of diet to reduce the amount of air ingested and to promote proper bowel function. Bloodworms and brine shrimp were on the menu.

I hoped Jeff would perk up and right himself after a suitable dietary change.

One of my next patients had an equally obvious problem but one that required a bit more intervention on my part. Barney was a springer spaniel. His happy face and furiously wagging tail told me those two parts of his body were fine, but as he hopped into the consulting room on three legs, it was clear that his right hind foot was not.

"He was playing in the garden yesterday," explained his worried owner, "charging round as usual with his friend. There was suddenly a yelp and the next thing he was holding his leg off the ground. He touches it to the floor occasionally, but it's mainly in the air."

I knelt on the floor and made my acquaintance, before starting to make my examination. When examining a lame leg, I always start at the bottom and work up. I wiggle each toe, squeeze each pad and feel between each digit, checking for nail injuries, thorns stuck in the foot or interdigital cysts. Then I check the bones of the toes and up to the hock, the equivalent of our ankle, where I also assess the lateral stability and the integrity of the ligaments.

The popliteal lymph node, behind the stifle is next. If this is enlarged it usually indicates infection lower down the limb. Then it is on to stifle manipulation – checking for cranial drawer and tibial thrust that might indicate ligament damage. At this point, Barney winced and turned around to look at his leg. There was a noticeable laxity in his joint. The cranial cruciate ligament appeared to have been ruptured, or at least seriously frayed – a classic injury for football players and active dogs alike. Poor Barney would need X-rays, painkillers and possibly surgery to correct this injury. There was so much more that I could do to help Barney – medicine and tests rather than bloodworms and brine shrimp!

Forty-Eight Hours in May

I was in the middle of another run. Nine nights out of ten on-call, either first or second. Normally, second-on-call means keeping a vigilant eye (or rather, an ear) out for the phone, either ringing or pinging to signify another pair of veterinary hands is needed. This is often for a difficult calving that requires a caesarean, but also can be for an operation (like the dog with a bladder tumour, that needed emergency surgery on Sunday night), or if two emergencies happen at the same time (like the horse with grass sickness that came in at exactly the same time as a calving).

Second-on-call is usually fairly quiet, but not so this week, as two of my nights on second were very busy. Both times my phone pinged into life just after midnight, a time when I am often fast asleep. Bank holiday Monday did not prove to be much of a holiday.

The series of WhatsApp messages told the story in increasing detail. *"C-section cow"* was the first message, swiftly followed by the name and address. Then more messages appeared as I fumbled for my clothes. *"2 front feet"*, *"2 hind feet"*, *"and a head"* told me that this was going to be a long night.

Four feet and a head means one of three things. It could be twins, all jumbled up. It could be one calf in a very odd presentation with all its limbs trying to exit the birth canal at the same time. Or worse, it could mean a deformed calf.

I shook myself awake and headed south, trying to steer a straight line and not fall asleep. It had been a busy weekend and I was already exhausted. A disturbed night's sleep and the prospect of a caesarean in the dark and the rain was the last thing I needed.

Candela was on first call and had already prepped the cow for surgery. I had a feel to see if there was any way the calf could be delivered naturally. The multitude of limbs was confusing and, more importantly, there was no way of manipulating them into a more sensible order. It would need to come out of the "side door" –

a phrase used by many experienced farmers to describe a caesarean section. Candela made the first incision. I pushed the legs back inside at the same time to make it easier.

But easy it was not. The limbs had no flexibility and could not be easily manoeuvred into position, making this one of the hardest caesareans I had done. We huffed and puffed, made our incision longer, pulled and pushed, until eventually the calf was out. It was very abnormal, with a horrible deformity called "schistosomus reflexus". Its legs were all wrong and its intestines hanging out. It wasn't alive but at least the cow was safe.

Forty-eight hours later, we were at it again. This time I headed north from the warmth of my bed, again just after midnight, again with Candela the unfortunate first-on-call vet. She was all set to go as soon as I arrived. The side of the cow was clipped and her flank was numbed, and Candela's head torch was in place.

"I'm terribly sorry, Julian," were her first words, full of apology for another disturbed night. But there was no need to apologise – she would have been even more tired than I was. Before I scrubbed my arm, my first job – the most important one of the evening – was to give my exhausted colleague a hug. We both needed it!

Within the hour, we had a healthy calf, a contented mum, a happy farmer and two delighted vets. We were exhausted, but the successful outcome made it all worthwhile!

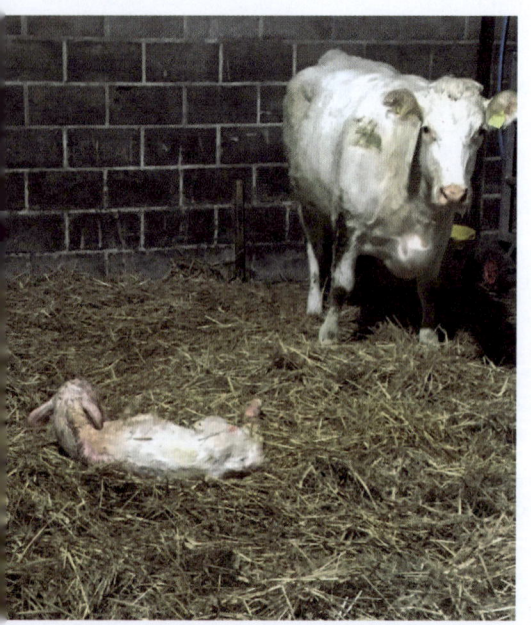

Hit the Hotspot

It was a simple case, although its name made it sound complicated. Moss the collie had acute superficial pyotraumatic dermatitis, a nasty but quite common condition in dogs. Its other name – "hotspot" – makes it sound much less serious, or like a good place to pick up free Wi-Fi. For a variety of reasons – a flea bite, a sore ear, a full and troublesome anal gland, or even just an itch – a dog will start to scratch. But instead of stopping once the itch has been relieved, the dog continues to scratch or lick and soon a minor irritation turns into a painful, infected mess oozing green pus. The end result of this concerted scratching is something much worse than it was at the start.

From the point of view of the vet, a hotspot is an easy thing to diagnose – there is no need for any blood tests, nor X-rays or scans. All we need is our eyes. And, for all they are a mess and a big problem, hotspots are quite straightforward to treat. The first job is to clip off the hair. Sticky, gooey hair stuck onto a painful lesion causes more soreness and removing it is a very important first step. It can be painful and sometimes we need to do this under sedation. Moss was a tolerant dog though, and stood patiently while I clipped. Once the hair is off the hotspot usually looks a lot less hot. It also looks much less like a spot, since the area can be much bigger than first impressions suggest.

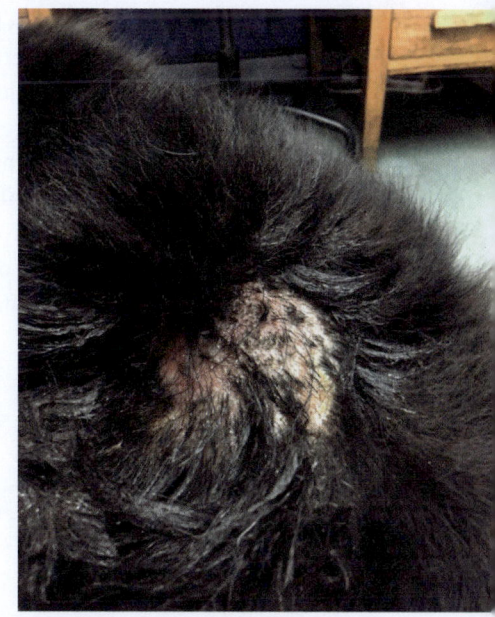

The next job is gentle bathing with warm water, antiseptic and cotton wool, cleaning away infected tissue and gunk. Once this is sorted out, the skin looks much more healthy. Some soothing gel, a course of antibiotics and sometimes anti-inflammatories to take away the soreness and remove the urge to itch, and the serious-benign condition with the fancy-not-so-fancy name is on its way to being fixed.

The final job is to try to find the cause of the original scratching. I search for fleas, check the anal glands and examine the ears. Sometimes there is no sign of what started it, and this was the case with Moss, but I knew that he would be feeling much, much better by the morning.

Another patient this week had an altogether different problem. It was my own dog, Emmy. Emmy is a picture of energetic health and, apart from the occasional accident – usually as a result of rushing around at high speed, without considering the consequences – she rarely needs veterinary attention. Emmy would follow me to the end of the earth (as long as I had a tennis ball) and she loves accompanying me on my calls and sitting in my car.

We were out for our usual morning walk – a high-speed excursion for her and an uninterrupted twenty minutes before the hectic challenges of the day for me. It was a lovely, sunny morning and Emmy was at full tilt. She had investigated all corners of Sowerby Flatts and made friends with owners, other dogs and the miscellaneous cattle which frequent these meadows. On our way back, she stopped to go to the toilet and I reached into my back pocket for the obligatory plastic bag. I bent down, be-bagged hand ready to scoop the poop. But what the heck was that, squirming and white and wiggling on the surface of the poo? Before my very eyes was a *tapeworm*! My own, healthy dog, wormed as regularly(ish) as she should be, was infested with parasites! I was mortified. Most urgent job, once I'd got to work: find my dog a wormer!

RTS Again

Last Friday, Anne and I put on our evening gear and headed to Leeds for the annual Royal Television Society awards. We were part of a huge contingent from Daisybeck Studios, the Leeds-based production company responsible for producing not only *The Yorkshire Vet*, but *Springtime on the Farm*, *Help the Animals at Christmas* and the *Britain's Favourite...* series, all of which had been nominated for awards. As we all descended on the Queen's Hotel, there was mounting excitement.

Over gin and tonics in the bar, the chatter was all about the chances of each of the nominees.

"Surely it's our turn this year?" I had been heard to say on more than one occasion. Hot money was on the *Britain's Favourite* series, although I suspected that *Help the Animals at Christmas* and *Springtime on the Farm* both had great chances of receiving a "gong". This was the fourth year in a row that *The Yorkshire Vet* had been nominated, this time in the category for "Best Documentary". We had been unsuccessful so far, so I had given up the idea of preparing an acceptance speech or even a list of people I must remember to thank. However, since we were nominated in two categories this year, the odds of a win had at least doubled. Based on sheer volume of episodes alone, we surely had to have a decent chance of bagging the prize. As the wine was poured and the starters arrived, I rummaged for my pen to jot down a few thoughts. Just in case. Paul Stead noticed this and came to offer some guidance: "If we win, Julian, just say a few words. Speak from your heart."

I needed to pace myself with the wine because, even if we didn't win, I would still be spending some time on the stage with my hands on a trophy. I'd been asked to present one of them; the award for "One to Watch". It was the penultimate prize, so I sipped at a slow and steady pace in case I dropped it, said the wrong thing (in my mind I had a plan to make a joke along the lines of: "And the winner is ... *La La Land*") or even fell off the stage.

But as the evening wore on, the tension started to rise and my resolution to maintain a sensible wine consumption weakened. Best Single Documentary, Best Presenter, Best Drama and Professional Excellence in Post Production all came and went with no prizes for Daisybeck. Everyone was getting more anxious but more excited and slightly more drunk.

Then came *The Yorkshire Vet*'s category: Best Documentary Series.

"And the winner is ... *THE YORKSHIRE VET!*" announced the host for the evening, the hilarious Reverend Kate Bottley.

An uproarious reaction erupted from the Daisybeck corner of the room. Amidst enthusiastic applause from the audience, we all trouped onto the stage to receive the award. It was emotional, for many reasons. Much of the team had been there from the very beginning over four years ago, and this was an important milestone we had reached together, all working very hard and pulling together. The passion and enthusiasm of Paul and his team, in particular the producer-directors with whom we, the vets, work so closely, has been infectious and tonight's award was the culmination of all that work. To be able to share what we do with anyone who cares to watch on a Tuesday night is reward in itself. Vets and nurses, owners and patients, get satisfaction from a happy outcome, but sharing this with one and a half million viewers is a wonderful thing. Winning an award is just the cherry on top.

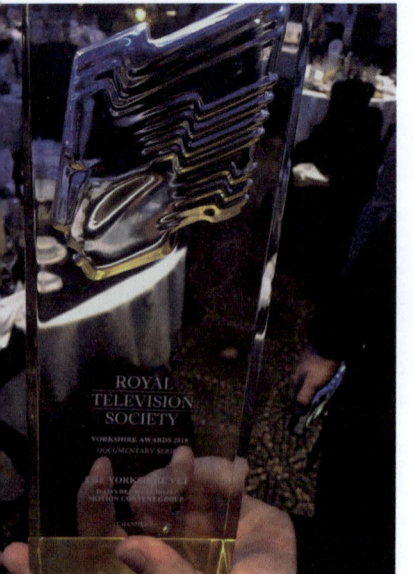

On stage, I realised I'd forgotten the notes I'd made, but it didn't matter. I spoke from the heart.

Princess with the Back End Injury

I took the opportunity at lunchtime to enjoy some late spring sunshine. After a morning in the consulting room I was in need of some fresh air and my dog, Emmy, needed a walk. Armed with my sandwich, a dog lead and a poo bag, we set off along the banks of the Ure. We could both have continued for much longer than lunchtime allowed, but there was enough time to sit down for a few minutes by the lock at Milby. I ate my sandwich while Emmy rummaged in the hedge, looking for adventures.

On the way back, we met a family – father, three children and their multiple dogs – as they headed out for an afternoon beside the river.

"Hello, Julian," exclaimed one of the young children. The familiarity of her tone suggested that we knew each other or, at least, had met before. Since every one of the four was wearing sunglasses, I didn't recognise them straightaway. The father lifted his sunglasses and explained: "It's a while since we've seen you – we are the bottom family!"

This was not so much help as you might think. I couldn't think of many friends who would describe themselves in such a way.

"Princess . . . from a year or two ago?"

This was the piece of information I required.

"Oh, yes, of course. I didn't recognise you with all these dogs!" I said, which was a reason as genuine as the sunglasses were an excuse.

Princess was a cat who I treated late in the summer of 2017. The accident-prone cat had been out doing what cats do, when major calamity befell her. She appeared back at home with the most enormous injury, extending under her tail, across her back legs and all around her sensitive and important bits. Nobody knew what had happened and I could not offer any explanation – it was an injury unlike any I had seen before.

Needless to say, I took her straight to theatre and embarked on what turned out to be pretty epic surgery, which took me late into the night. Perineal reconstruction is a fiddly thing, but the surgery went well and, after an hour or so, Princess looked almost as good as new – or at least, all the bits were back in the right places. I was really pleased with how it had come together, and I knew that when Princess woke from her anaesthetic she would be a lot happier. The third delighted person that evening was Laura, my camera girl at the time.

"Julian, that was totally amazing. Thank you for letting me film it!" she said, brimming with enthusiasm, before giving me a hug and rushing off to save the exciting footage on a hard drive somewhere. It would be a strong story for one of the later episodes of series five of *The Yorkshire Vet*. On this sunny afternoon by the river, that seemed like a lifetime ago.

"And how is she getting on?" I asked. The last time I had seen her, the injury was healing spectacularly well, as much due to the powers of the body to repair itself as to my painstaking suture placement, I suspected. But I hadn't seen her since then and I hoped that not only had her wounds healed completely, but also, given the mangling their external orifices had received, her bowel and bladder function was intact.

"She's fine, completely healed and back to normal," enthused the father. "You'd never have known there had been a problem. We were so pleased you fixed her. That reminds me. One of our dogs has a problem with his anal glands. We must bring him in to see you. We know you're an expert down there!"

Nelly with Legs Like an Elephant

Anne and I had been treating Nelly for over a year. Anne had removed a lump from the feisty little Scottie's toe. Analysis of the growth had shown it to be a nasty tumour, so I saw her regularly to check it wasn't re-growing. She had been doing very well and we dared to hope that she had made a full recovery. However, a month or so ago, things took a turn for the worse. She developed some vague, non-specific signs of illness – gummy eyes and a reluctance to go for her usual walks. Then, a strange thing started to happen. Her legs started to get fatter. It was subtle at first and just affecting the front legs, but by the time I'd arranged for her to come in for X-rays to investigate, it was very obvious.

I was concerned it might be a condition called Hypertrophic Pulmonary Osteopathy, or Marie's disease. This is a bizarre syndrome whereby the bones of the front (and sometimes also the back) legs become thickened, as a result of a mass of some description growing in the lungs. Nobody seems to know exactly why this happens and it is pretty rare, but is something I always consider when I see a dog like this. I explained my concerns. X-rays of the legs and also the chest would confirm or rule out the problem.

The X-rays were conclusive. Nelly did, indeed, have legs like an elephant. The cortices of the bones in her front legs and feet were distended and irregular. The chest X-rays also showed more bad news. There was an obvious, plum-sized mass sitting slap bang in the centre of the right lung lobe. I called with the grave news.

"What can we do?" was the next question.

Steroids would help. I prescribed a course and they worked wonders for a time, but then the signs started to return. At this point, surgery to remove the lung lobe containing the tumour seemed the only option left. It was serious surgery, not for the faint-hearted and without any guarantee of success. After some further discussion, we all agreed it was worth the risk. If the surgery went well Nelly could be cured. Without it, she couldn't continue. When put in such bleak terms, the decision seemed simple and we arranged a time for the operation.

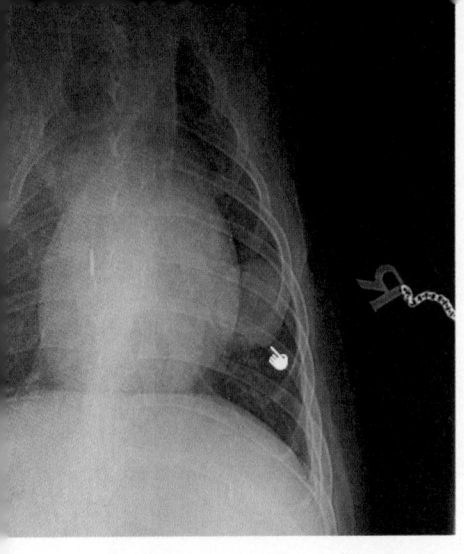

A thoracotomy and lung lobectomy was pencilled in for the following week and big stars were placed all over the day book to alert nurses and reception staff not to arrange any other procedures for the same day.

Not many lung tumours are amenable to surgery. Most of them spread rampantly through the lung tissue with secondaries seeded everywhere. They are usually associated with serious breathing problems and the prognosis following intervention can be terrible. But Nelly was different – her lung tumour was not actually affecting her respiratory system at all. Just her painful, elephantine legs and her disposition.

It was all hands on deck. Anne was there to help with the surgery, while two nurses dealt with the anaesthetic – not only did Nelly need to stay asleep, but also her lungs needed to be ventilated manually all the time we were inside the chest. The tumour was sitting there, just as it appeared on the X-ray, circumscribed and red, right in the middle of the lung lobe. My plan was to remove the whole lobe.

As I placed the final sutures across the lung tissue, sealing the airways so I could remove the tumour, I said, "It's just like that song by CamelPhat".

Of course I meant the recent one called "Breath" rather than the previous one called "Panic Room".

Cute Puppy with a Strange Eye

Nelly, the Scottie dog with the lung tumour, made a spectacular recovery from her surgery. She went home later the same day and never looked back. At a follow-up appointment a few days later, her owners were effusive.

"It's a miracle. She's like a puppy again. Thank you so much!"

Over subsequent check-ups, we measured her legs using a tape measure. Sure enough, the firm swellings around her toes and long bones gradually reduced in circumference. Removal of the offending lung tumour had reversed the bony proliferation that was characteristic of the syndrome called Hypertrophic Pulmonary Osteopathy from which Nelly was suffering. It was as if, like Alice, she had imbibed the contents of a bottle with the words *"drink me"* on the label. Her legs shrunk back down to normal proportions and her demeanour was restored almost immediately. It was an amazing case.

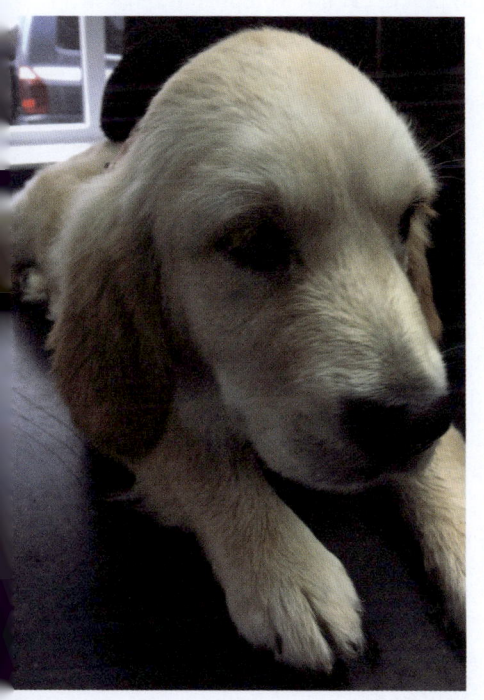

Another condition I saw that same week was much more perfunctory, but no less problematic for the dog and its owners.

Harriet was a young and very cute golden retriever puppy. As she sauntered into the consulting room, her anxious owners explained that they had noticed a strange swelling in the corner of one of her eyes, concluding: "We've never seen anything like it!"

Luckily though, I had. Unlike Nelly's problem, which was

pretty rare, Harriet's condition was very common. It also had a much more benign sounding name. Harriet had a "cherry eye". Cherry eye is a pretty accurate description of the appearance of the swelling near the lower side of the inside corner of the eye, although it is never quite as big as a cherry. Neither is the swelling quite the same colour as a cherry. "Redcurrant eye" would be a better term. It is more properly described as "prolapse of the third eyelid (or nictitans) gland". This is a gland that produces tears and it lives (when it is in its normal position) behind the third eyelid. The third eyelid is, as the name suggests, a third eyelid, in addition to the upper and lower eyelids, and it acts as a protective mechanism for dogs and cats who rush into bushes and hedges without thinking about what might happen to their eyes. Behind it is a tear gland which helps to keep the eyes hydrated and lubricated. For some reason, this gland can pop out of its normal position and stick out from behind the third eyelid, just like a cherry. Well, more like a redcurrant.

I examined the eye, which was very simple and straightforward and explained the problem and what was required. Once it is out of position, the gland never stays in place, even if you push it back in, and surgical intervention is required. In the past, vets would simply chop it off and the offending blob would miraculously disappear. Nowadays, it is generally thought that this isn't a great idea, since it reduces the amount of tear producing tissue, which can cause issues later in life. If possible, we try to replace it, restoring normal function, improving the abnormal appearance and removing any chance of damage to the prolapsed gland.

I arranged to see Harriet later in the week for the appropriate surgery. Her owners were worried, but Harriet was not. Her last trip to the vets, after all, had been very pleasant, without any nasty injections and not even a thermometer. She trotted in with enthusiasm to see me. I fussed her fluffy head and reassured her and her owners that all would be good. And all was good. Harriet recovered nicely, her eye back to normal. I would see her again a few days later and there would be no requirement for a tape measure.

Burton Leonard

I had an important engagement after I'd finished morning surgery the Saturday before last. I had been co-opted by Stray FM radio presenter Will Smith, to be the judge at the fancy dress competition at Burton Leonard Feast. Will has been very helpful promoting stuff to do with *The Yorkshire Vet*, so I felt I owed him a favour, but I also love these traditional village events – this one dates back to the 1850s. As I was on duty, beeper permitting, I would be in the area during the afternoon. If I were to get a call, it wasn't far to the surgery to stitch up an injured dog, or administer cortisone to a cat stung by a bee.

So, the horse with conjunctivitis had been treated, phone calls had been made to discuss lab results and the last consultation of the morning (a rat with an infection) had been completed. Next Stop: Burton Leonard. The first time I ever encountered this village was when I ran in their 10K race, about as many years ago. Now, I go through the village every week – I was there on Monday, pregnancy testing cows and heifers. Saturday's job, however, would be very different – no plastic, arm-length gloves, no wellies and no cows – but still all eyes would be on me as I pronounced my decision. It wasn't "pregnant" or "not pregnant" but ". . . and the winner is . . ."

We all processed down the road, stopping the traffic, to tunes from Knaresborough brass band, before arriving at the Fancy Dress Show Ring. The first few classes were exciting enough: The Barbara Iveson Trophy, a veritable jug if ever there was one, went to the winner of *The Best Dressed Pram* category. There were not so many entries into the *Decorated Bike* category (I suspected most cyclists were taking advantage of a warm, sunny Saturday and actually riding their bikes), but it got better with Mr Potatohead taking third prize in the next category, which was for *Girls and Boys 2 Years and Under*.

There was a surprise for me in the *Girls and Boys 5 and 6 Years* category, as one contestant came dressed as me, complete with checked shirt, stethoscope and my first book (*Horses, Heifers and Hairy Pigs: The Life of a Yorkshire Vet*, still available in all good bookshops). Not surprisingly, he won. After all the age group classes, up to and including *Ladies and Gents*, the *Open Couples* category came along. Now, as an outsider to the village, I had no idea what this class might entail, and my mind boggled slightly, particularly when an assistant sitting nearby whispered in my ear, "This one is for the mad people."

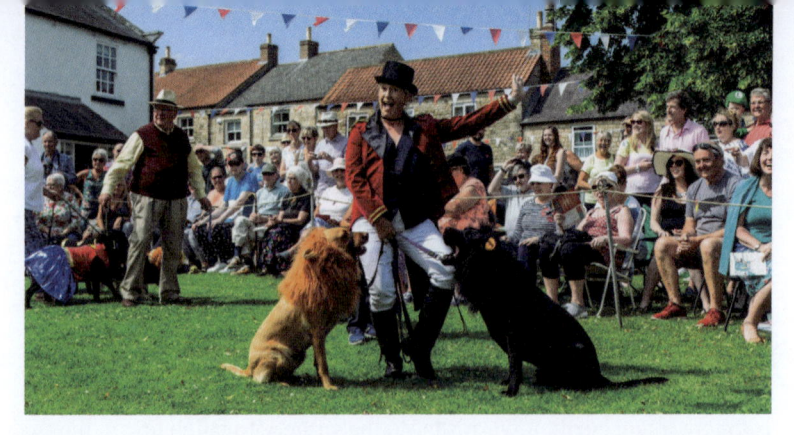

The first two contestants were dressed as exact replicas of Mr and Mrs Green, of *Yorkshire Vet* fame. Their outfits, complete with floral dress and trainers, were perfect and their rendition was completed with a running commentary as they did a lap of the ring.

As if this wasn't sufficient excitement for the day, the final class was a new category, specially introduced this year: *The Best Dressed Pet*. In a popular and closely fought class, Batman (a dachshund) and Robin (a basset hound) were narrowly beaten by a pair of lions. I relaxed with an ice-cream for a few moments and then my phone rang. It was back into veterinary action – a Labrador pup had eaten some poisonous berries. At last I was back into familiar territory.

But not for long!

In just a few days I would be at another show – one that was just a bit bigger – in Harrogate. I would be out of my comfort zone again, up an eighty-foot pole and back on telly. But more of that next week . . .

The Great Yorkshire Show

"Julian, how do you feel about climbing a pole at the Great Yorkshire Show?"

It wasn't the usual type of question, but Emily was busy planning the filming schedule for Channel 5's programme *Today at The Great Yorkshire Show*.

I had got to know Emily while she was working on *The Yorkshire Vet* and she was a good friend. I could trust her completely and so, even though what she was suggesting had shades of the scene in *Bridget Jones*, when Bridget was filmed from an unfortunate angle sliding down a fireman's pole, I felt I was probably in safe hands.

"OK, go on then," I replied, with only a very slight hesitation, "if you think it will be a good thing."

My inner competitor already had me rising to the challenge. I had climbed lots of things in the past – many rock faces at Brimham Rocks, Scugdale and Almscliffe. I had been to the top of near vertical ice faces in the Scottish mountains in winter and I had climbed the steep sides of many Alps, both with ice-axes and rock-climbing kit and on skis. How hard could an eighty-foot tree trunk be?

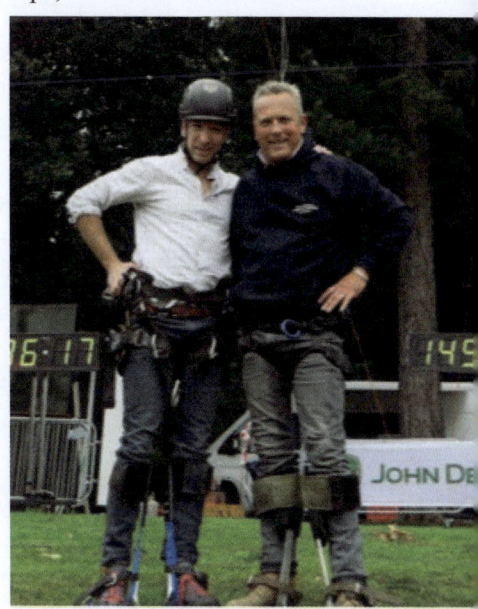

But without any practising whatsoever and with a huge crowd watching (and also a crowd of about 1.6 million viewers as it would turn out the following evening on Channel 5), I felt strangely apprehensive as I donned my harness and the specially designed spikes which tree climbers wear for their work. We watched one of the pros run up the huge pole like a mountain goat, sprinting to the top in a mere ten seconds. Then it was our turn.

I wished Jules (Hudson) good luck. He was outwardly chipper, but obviously just as anxious as I was and probably further outside of his zone of comfort. But he was a proper TV presenter and must have done this sort of thing many times before. I thought about the classic *Blue Peter* feature from the 1970s, when John Noakes climbed up Nelson's Column by means of a wooden ladder. Today should, at least, be a safer proposition than that heroic exploit. We shook hands (or did we pump fists like successful batsmen, I can't remember?) and then waited for the starting whistle.

It was hard at first, mainly because I could not find a rhythm, but also because it was vertical. I fumbled, slipped and cursed that I had not had the chance to practise at all. Surely, I would not be humiliated on my home turf of Yorkshire and on national telly? I glanced across to see Jules several feet ahead of me, relaxed and in a rhythm. I looked up – it was miles to the top. I looked down – I had not progressed far.

But with gritted teeth, I somehow managed to get to the top of the pole, which was swaying vigorously with both the breeze and from the movements of my climbing. It took me 86 seconds, versus 149 seconds for my competitor and my fellow presenter. I was happy to have made it to the top first, although I would have liked to go sub sixty seconds. Maybe next year?

In the meantime, we had another TV interview to do. Then there was book-signing, a radio interview and an appointment with a farrier, who was going to teach me how to make a horseshoe. I really wanted to head over to the cattle classes – they all look so magnificent and I'd promised to call and see some old friends. I never did make it, nor did I get to survey the sheep – at least not in any detail: I had seen them from the top of my pole! It had been the most hectic Yorkshire Show of all; but it had definitely been one of the best!

The Curious Incident of
the Dog on Sunday Morning

Gemma the Labrador came off worse in the skirmish that occurred on her Sunday morning walk. What was described over the telephone as a small gash on her shoulder turned out to be a large gash that would certainly need stitching. The teeth of Gemma's usually best friend had left a flap of skin that I would need to debride to give the wound a decent chance of healing. Dog-bite injuries tend to be complicated by squashed, bruised and devitalised tissue, so they need to be treated correctly.

I explained to her owners that surgery would be required and what was involved. By coincidence, Gemma's injury was almost identical to the one sustained by my cousin's Labrador the previous weekend, while my cousin was away (meeting up with us) and her daughter was in charge. She had messaged me about the dog's treatment and, more contentiously, the size and extent of the invoice, which ran to two sides of A4.

But for now, the Labrador in front of me was my priority. I sedated her, clipped and cleaned the wound and injected some local anaesthetic before debriding the damaged skin and putting in some sutures. I injected her with antibiotics and pain relief and took a few moments to admire a tidy, clean wound before finding a phone to call her owners.

They weren't far away, which was ideal. I reversed her sedation so she would be awake enough to walk to the car when they arrived. It had been successful and efficient and I could move on to my next job of the day.

As I typed the details into the computer, I scrolled back through the messages on my phone to the photo of the bill for my cousin's dog. It was nearly five times the amount I had charged for Gemma and full of extras: *1x dog GA* (obviously not an extra), *1x emergency operation surcharge* (I didn't have this on my bill), *1x suture wound dog moderate* (more than twice as much as mine), *7x additional 10 minutes* (70 minutes in addition to the suturing wound time). There were others too, *1x surgical instrumentation, 3x suture materials, 1x surgical cap, 1x surgical gown, 1x surgical drape, 1x flush wound major*. There was no wonder the invoice extended to two pages.

It raises an interesting point. Vets are skilled professionals and our salary should reflect this. At the moment there is a huge exodus of vets from the profession. Poor pay, long hours, and disillusionment with the corporate take-over of the profession giving few opportunities to progress, are just some of the contributing factors. I have just worked three nights on call and over a weekend, going straight into a full week including two nights on duty. The finances of mixed practice do not allow for sufficient veterinary staff to enable everyone to have Monday and Tuesday off after a weekend on call. So, maybe practice like the one where I work should be charging more?

But adding surcharges to a bill for items and procedures that are integral to the process is like adding a washing-up surcharge to a restaurant bill, plus an extra charge for the washing-up liquid. The bill of nearly *five times* my own came from one of the largest veterinary groups in the country, where surely at least some economies of scale should be passed to the clients, rather than to the CEOs with large watches and smooth suits.

The Labrador gets similar treatment, but the credit card of the owner takes the extra hit, or the insurance companies, who must be feeling squeezed, if not to say ripped off. Their response? Premiums go up, excesses rise and co-payments are added making insurance unaffordable. And for many, without insurance, these veterinary fees are also unaffordable. Meanwhile, the veterinary governing bodies sit on their hands oblivious to (or choosing to ignore) the huge disparity in fees between practices. Sadly, it does little to promote the image of veterinary practice to the general public.

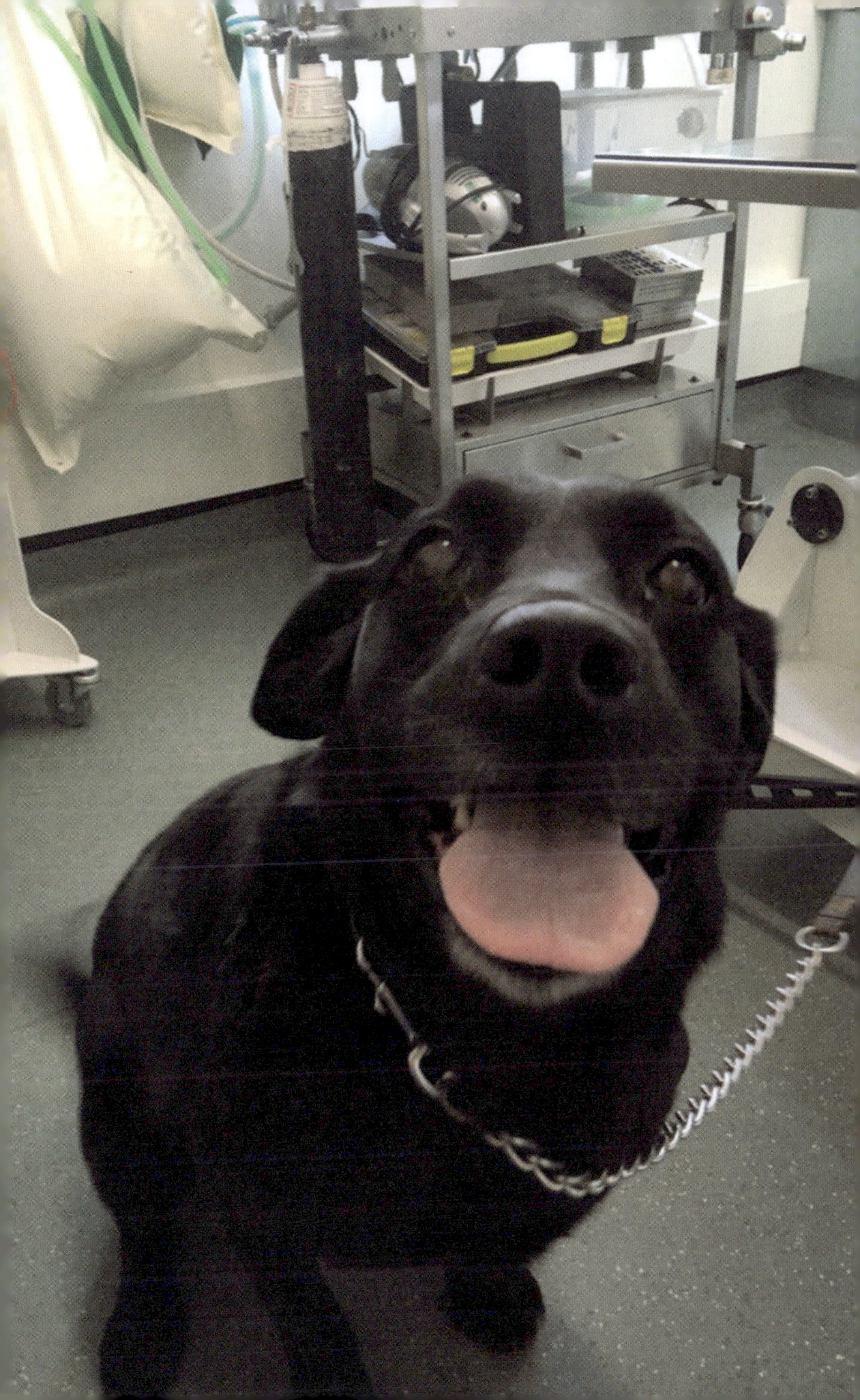

This week I Have Been Mostly Sticking My Finger Up Dogs' Bums

This week I have been mostly sticking my finger up dogs' bums. It sounds like a line from an episode of *The Fast Show* with Jesse the tramp, played by the hilarious Mark Williams. But it is actually quite true. Not for fun, mind you. There are a multitude of reasons why a vet needs to do this and the donning of a latex glove, followed by the liberal application of gloopy lubricant to the index finger is an act with which all veterinarians are well acquainted. It is not a very nice thing for the dog, nor for the vet, but it is necessary to investigate and treat all sorts of problems – prostate disease, hernias, growths and masses and, of course, the dreaded anal glands. These noxious structures are scent glands, which sit on either side of the anus, at approximately four o'clock and eight o'clock, if you imagine the anus as a clock face (don't dwell on the image though). These glands fill up with a horrible, smelly secretion, which usually empties when dogs pass faeces, to act as a method of marking territory. Since dogs' territory is usually marked nowadays by the garden fence or the perimeter of the park around which they are taken for their morning walk, the glands are largely redundant and a nuisance rather than of any benefit.

Sometimes they don't empty properly and the result can be *impaction of the anal glands*, which sounds like a condition from pre-Herriot days. The finger is inserted to allow palpation of each gland. It is easy to tell if the gland is full – there is no need for complicated tests or MRI scans to diagnose the problem and, in any case, even before we insert the lubricated digit, the behaviour of the dog as described by its owner is usually enough to identify the problem.

"He's been scooting along the ground and going mad with his back end," is a common description. "She can't stop licking under her tail," is another. Either way, it is easy to identify impacted glands and also easy to fix. Squeezing the left gland and then the right and mopping up or catching all of the smelly contents in a wodge of cotton wool is one of the first things that vets learn to do and one of the first jobs that senior vets delegate to juniors and that junior vets delegate to students.

I can remember exactly my first encounter with the anal glands of a dog. I was an enthusiastic school boy, eager to become a vet one day. I would walk to the local vets in Castleford after school and spend a few hours watching, learning and helping out (to a small extent – there was not very much useful that a school child could do, but I tried to get as much practical experience as possible). Thursday evenings were long but full of interest and excitement and I would always get home, well after eight, with aching feet from standing up, hungry for my tea and thirsty for more knowledge. In the case of the anal gland encounter, I was just a bit too thirsty for knowledge as I leaned in, peering under the dog's tail to get a better view. The vet, clearly without concern for the vet-to-be, gave not a hint of a warning as he squeezed the foul-smelling glands. A fountain of stinking, fetid liquid paste splattered my face, into my mouth and all over my hair. I tried to maintain my composure in this most horrible of circumstances. But it stood me in good stead for the future. I treat the anal area of dogs with a healthy respect and I ALWAYS warn students if their enthusiasm takes them just a bit too close!

Bull's Eye, Owl's Eye

My first visit had already been arranged when I arrived at work on Wednesday morning. It wasn't at all what I expected.

"There's a farmer who wants you to take his bull's eye out."

The message was unequivocal and it put a small spanner in the workings of my day, which was already pretty full. I made a few phone calls to rearrange my morning and headed out with armfuls of surgical equipment, lots of local anaesthetic and some trepidation. It is not a common operation to undertake and I had only done the procedure on cattle twice before.

The first time didn't go too well. It was complicated by an extensive tumour that was growing from the unfortunate Simmental's third eyelid and proved impossible to remove. The second time, the op went perfectly, which was just as well because it was all being filmed for *The Yorkshire Vet*. The bull in question had a huge, swollen, glaucomatous eye and the farmer was, quite rightly, worried it might pop. It must have been painful, although the young bull in question appeared stoically normal. Aptly, the condition of a hugely swollen eye is called *buphthalmos*, which derives from the Greek and literally means "ox eye". I hoped this third occasion would go as smoothly as the last.

When I got to the farm, the animal whose eye I was instructed to remove, did not look so stoic as my previous patient. The eye, however, did look terrible and there was surely no hope of the injury healing naturally. There had been some kind of accident – the spikey, thorny type of accident, which is not good for the delicate structures of the eyeball. So, as you might expect, the eyeball had come off worse. The injury had gone undetected for a day or so and the topical ointment the farmer had applied had not proved very effective.

I agreed that the only way forwards, to alleviate the pain and to have any chance of healing, was to remove the eye. Once the head was restrained, I clipped off all the hair and then instilled as much local anaesthetic as I could. There are some specific nerves that we aim for, with a long needle. The local will numb the nerve and provide perfect analgesia. However, it is hard to find the exact location of these nerves and so it is sensible to inject as much local as is possible. Finally, the whole op site was numb and I set about the (rather basic) surgery. Half an hour later the final suture was in place, the eye was out and the outcome was pretty good. I stood up, stretched out my aching back and admired my work. The bullock seemed oblivious to what had just happened, although maybe just a bit confused about the numbness to the right side of his face. It must have been like a very serious trip to the dentist for an extraction, albeit a rather different sort of extraction.

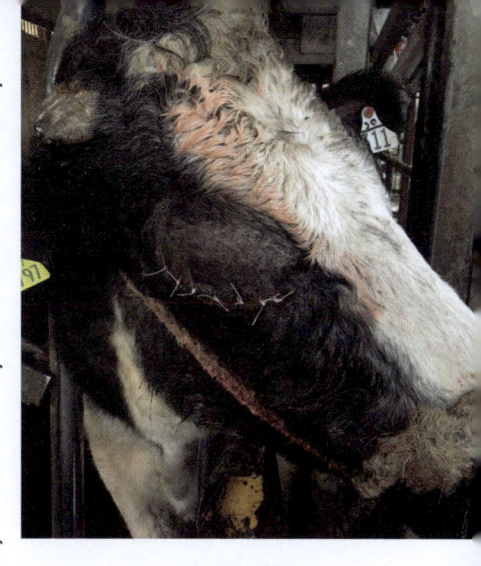

I cleaned up and headed off to continue my rounds, leaving a happy patient and a grateful farmer, and feeling satisfied.

Later, back at the practice, I ticked my way through a list of phone calls. The last one involved an owl.

"Julian, thanks for calling me back," said Joe, answering my call. Joe kept a selection of unusual creatures and owls were part of his menagerie.

"I've got this owl and I'm worried about his eye," he explained. "It's badly ulcerated and I've been putting drops in, but it's no better. I think it needs to be removed. Can I book it in?"

It was my turn to roll my eyes, skywards this time. This would be even harder!

Grass Seed in Eye

After the excitement of both a bullock and an owl with a troublesome eye last week, this week it was the turn of a dog to receive my ophthalmological attention. Barney was a spaniel and if his health was to be judged by the ferocious wagging of his tail, then it would be assumed that he was completely healthy. However, a closer inspection at the other end of his body revealed a big problem.

"I think he's got conjunctivitis," explained his owner. "It's been like it for a day or so and it's not getting any better, so that's why he's here."

Barney did not want to stay still, so it wasn't very easy to examine him in a lot of detail. However, his left eye was clearly very sore, running with gooey, greenish-yellow pus as well as a watery discharge. It was almost closed, but the bit that could be seen showed a scarlet red inflammation of the inner membranes.

I already had a pretty good idea of what might be going on and asked a few questions about the onset of the problem.

"Well, he'd been running through a field – as he does – and it was soon after that when it started. I wonder if there could be some dust or pollen in it?"

I suspected the problem was something a bit bigger than specks of pollen and immediately reached for a little vial of anaesthetic eye drops. Once the drops had been trickled in, everything became easier as Barney's pain eased and the spasm in his eyelids relaxed. This allowed me to examine him properly. Under the third eyelid there was the tell-tale brownish speck which suggested a grass seed. Grass seeds are a common problem in summer time and a problem to which spaniels seem particularly prone. I think it's a combination of their height – just the same as the long grass through which they rummage – and also the way that they spring and bounce through the fields. Whatever the reason, Barney certainly had one in his eye. I explained my plan to Barney's owner, who didn't seem to understand quite what I was saying ("A grass seed in his eye? How can that be?" I could imagine, in the thought bubble hovering above his head).

With artery forceps, I carefully everted the third eyelid to allow me a closer look underneath. There it was. Only its spikey end was visible, but it was definitely there. I carefully grabbed the end I could see and let Barney pull backwards, so that the foreign body emerged.

It was just as I expected – a seed of grass, complete with head, long tail and irritating barbs. It was out of his eye and in the teeth of my forceps. Grass seeds are the enemy of vets during the summer. Because of their pointed sharp tip and their barbed structure, they only travel in one direction – inwards. They commonly poke into the space between the toes and migrate upwards. I've even seen them pierce the skin of the foot and work their way all the way up to pop out in the armpit.

If a grass seed gets inhaled (again, typically in enthusiastic springer spaniels who suck in extra air to fuel their vigorous summer activities) it can end up in the lungs and the outcome is really bad as it scrapes its way through the delicate tissue of the lungs. Repeated bouts of pneumonia develop and havoc is reeked.

But Barney was easily fixed, without the pesky seed penetrating further inside his body. Painful and troublesome as a seed in the eye must have been, now it was out, and with a tube or two of ointment, Barney would be completely fine.

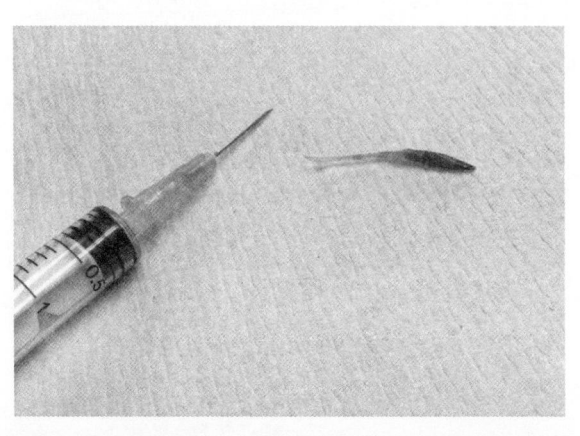

Just Chuck it up, Duck

Perky had been with us for a couple of days and already had made himself comfortable in a quiet corner of the kennels. Perky wasn't his real name, but his only other form of identification was the number on the ring on his leg. It didn't seem very nice to refer to this racing pigeon simply by his number, so we hit upon Perky as an apt name. But while Perky *was* fairly perky, he was not really very good at racing. He'd been found by a passer-by, sitting on a village green just outside Boroughbridge. Many tourists had been doing a similar thing over the warm summer, some having travelled long distances to get here. We did not know where Perky's journey had started, but it must have been a long way away, because he was tired, hungry and dehydrated when he was brought into the vets.

The lost pigeon was just one of the waifs and strays under our care at the time. At the opposite end of the kennels was a hedgehog who had been found, equally bewildered and in a place where he shouldn't have been, out and about during the daytime. Just like a racing pigeon sitting on the village green, a hedgehog who is out in the daytime is clearly in trouble and it was right that he had been brought in for veterinary attention. The hedgehog had been given the name Horace, after the 1980s computer character, Hungry Horace, who crossed roads, avoiding traffic and trying to find things to eat. Horace the hedgehog had narrowly avoided a similar fate to his computer game namesake, and once we'd had chance to check him over, the spikey character's problems were very evident. Horace was covered in ticks, each one the size and shape of a piece of sweetcorn, full of the little hedgehog's blood which the horrible parasites had been sucking to engorge themselves, before detaching and laying lots of eggs. The result was severe anaemia for Horace. Every tick needed painstakingly to be removed.

After half an hour with the forceps, Horace was looking and feeling much better. He was free of ticks and the base of the kidney dish next to him was covered in the annoyed arachnids. We put him back to bed, with a bowl of cat food and some water. He would make a full recovery.

Perky the pigeon was also gaining strength. He had been eating and drinking well and looked altogether healthier. We'd even managed to find his owner by tracking his phone number via the identification number on his leg.

Sally, one of the nurses, called the owner to pass on the good news that we had found his pigeon, and find out what he wanted us to do with him. I guessed the owner might not be so excited, because a pigeon that didn't return home was surely not a very good homing pigeon. There was a possibility that he wouldn't want him back at all.

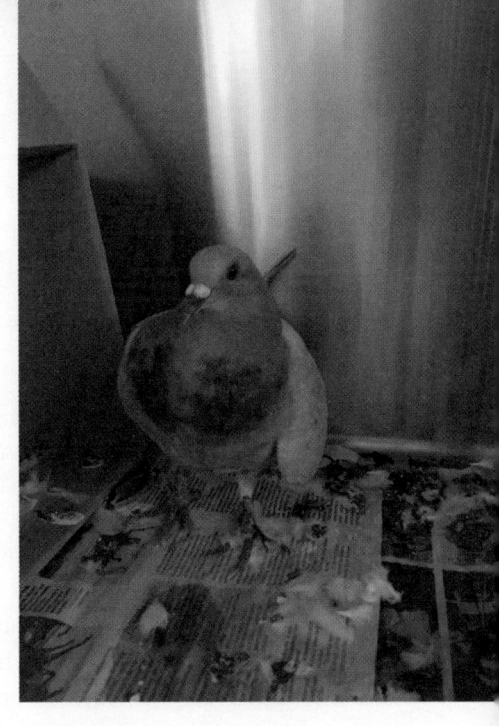

After several abortive attempts, Sally eventually managed to make contact. To our relief, Perky's owner was pleased his missing pigeon had been found and delighted that it had regained strength after a period of rest.

So, asked Sally, what should we do with Perky?

"Just chuck it up, duck!" were the instructions from the owner, who told us he was based in Derbyshire (although the suffix of "duck" was enough to tell us that the pigeon hailed from that part of the country!).

After morning ops had been finished, we took Perky outside and found a space clear of roads and traffic. He'd had a good drink and some breakfast and we held our breath and "chucked it up".

Betty

I had an important job to do after afternoon surgery on Friday. It was a visit, but not a visit to see a poorly animal. I had received a message from a friend who worked in a care home. They had a new resident, an old acquaintance of mine, whose dogs and guinea pigs I had looked after some years ago. Since then she had left her little bungalow, I had moved to a new practice and we had lost touch.

Betty had, unknowingly, become famous on the Internet because of her appearance in an early episode of *The Yorkshire Vet*, with her little dog, Billy. Billy, a laconic Shih Tzu, was a regular visitor to the surgery as a consequence of his tendency to eat the meals-on-wheels, which arrived at Betty's house every day. Tasty as these prepared meals were, they did not suit the little dog's bowels so well. The result was intermittent diarrhoea, which would often get stuck to Billy's fur, necessitating cleaning and clipping by me. It was a messy job, but one which I didn't mind, because it would give instant relief to Billy. Betty was always pleased with the problem solved. She was an amusing lady and was always glad of some human conversation, rather than the usual company of her dogs.

On that famous day, I'd seen Betty's name and Billy's name on the appointment list, followed by the words *growth on chest*. I knew she would be worried.

When I lifted Billy onto the table, the lump was easy to find. It was quite big – an inch or so long and maybe half an inch across.

"So, this lump, Betty. How long do you think it's been here?" I asked.

"I've only just noticed it," she replied. This was concerning. For a lump of this size only to have been detected recently, it must have grown very quickly. Slow growing masses are usually identified at a much smaller stage. The lump was also very attached to the skin and was covered in matted hair, suggesting it was discharging and therefore ulcerated or cystic. The matted hair made it very hard to inspect in detail so I started cautiously trimming hair away from the structure, to allow a more detailed examination.

As I snipped away, it started to dawn on me that this might not be a cancerous growth at all. Suddenly, a minty smell started to emanate from the mass and my fingers became sticky. The mass on Billy's chest was actually a boiled sweet! It had glued itself to his fur and, presumably, the more he tried to lick it off, the stickier it became. I related the good news to Betty. "It's a sweet, Mrs Taylor. It's just a sweet. I'd have felt a complete idiot if I'd anaesthetised little Billy, only to surgically remove a sweet!"

The relief was tangible on Betty's face. "It's a sweetie! Poor Billy! How did that get there, I wonder? And I thought it would need an operation! It's just a sweetie, stuck under his tummy!" We both fell around laughing, in relief and amusement!

The outcome was fortunate for everyone concerned, especially camera operator, Laura, who had been filming the whole, hilarious incident. The editors and post-production team would be just as delighted with the outcome. Not only did we enjoy the moment, but so did over three million others!

Needless to say, Betty was surprised to see me when I arrived late this Friday afternoon at the old people's home where she now lived. I was glad to see her, too. We chatted, reminiscing over her little dogs and especially Billy and the sweetie stuck to his tummy!

A photograph of one of my favourite patients, bringing back happy memories for us both.

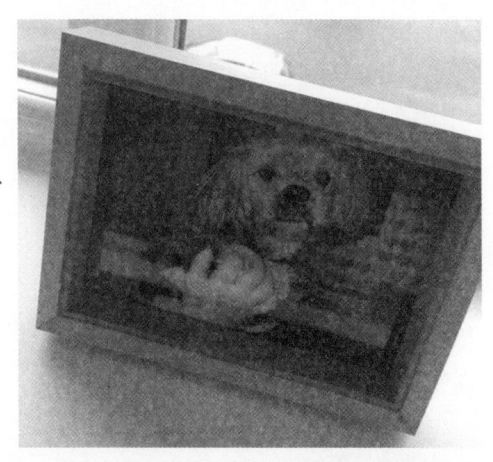

There's a Goose, Loose in the Lane

The extra appointment on my morning's list caught my attention:

"Two geese, injured by dogs."

It sounded more interesting than the two dogs with diarrhoea, the two Labradors with conjunctivitis and the couple of cats in need of their annual vaccinations. To see one goose was unusual, but to see two of these curious creatures was cause to make a call to my cameraman.

"Ross, there are two geese coming to see me later this morning. They have some injuries, but I don't know a lot more than that," I explained to Ross the cameraman, who was preparing to head out to follow up some cattle from a previous story.

He quickly changed his plans and rearranged his morning to come and meet the geese. And it was a good thing he did, because the pair of birds, a female and a gander, were soon sitting calmly and serenely in the waiting room. One was in a cardboard box, wearing one of those close-fitting outfits that babies wear. The other was in a laundry basket, with a pillow case over his head.

I called them in, or rather I called in their owner and immediately realised I would need to help carry them into the consultation room.

It transpired that the pair of terriers who lived on the farm, employed mainly to control the rat population, had taken a liking to (or rather, a vendetta against) the geese. The two of them had made an unfortunate attack on the birds. On this occasion, the birds had come off worse. Most dogs would steer well clear of a couple of belligerent geese, but the pair of Borders had obviously egged one another on. The result was some nasty injuries to both goose and gander. The terriers, on the other hand, were unscathed but (quite literally) in the dog house.

I examined the male goose first, carefully removing the pillowcase from his head. It wasn't so much that he was a hostage, being

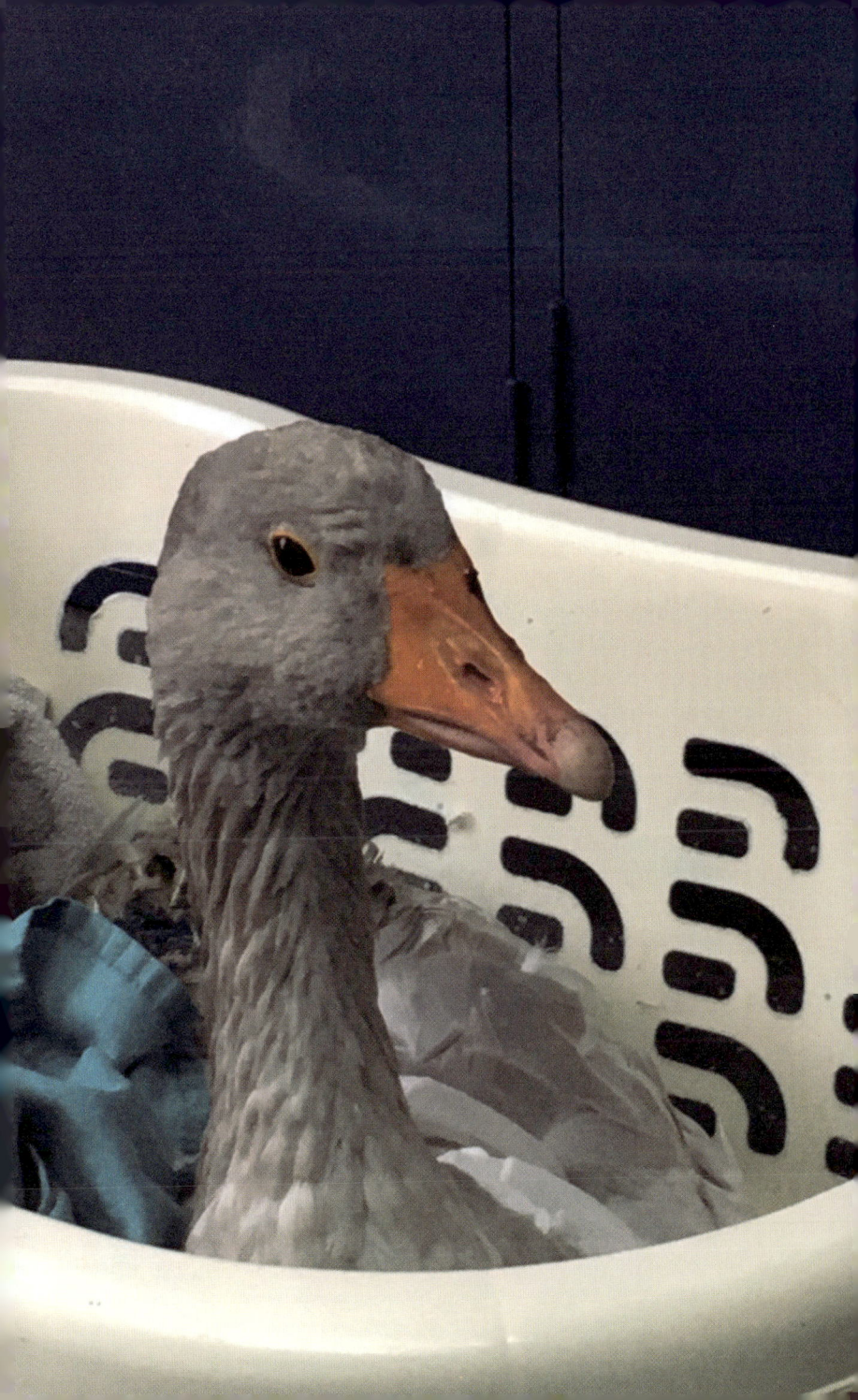

smuggled away from the scene by the goose police – rather, a pillow case over the head keeps a bird calm when in unfamiliar surroundings (a car journey to the vet's, for example) and it also keeps the snappy beak away from farmer's and vet's fingers. A large sock also works well.

His handsome face showed not a trace of illness as he looked around, checking out things to peck at. The large wound, which was obvious on his back, was where he had borne the brunt of the terrier attack. The female bird had similar injuries.

There was a lot of bruising, damage to the skin and some tissue necrosis, which is common with crushing injuries. Worst of all, fly eggs and little maggots had appeared in the dead and damaged tissue. It took a painstaking twenty minutes to rid Mr and Mrs Goose of all the maggots we could find. It is a grim, but strangely satisfying job, and all vets have their favoured technique. My personal favourite is using forceps to get the obvious ones. I then spray blue spray into the wound. The horrible grubs soon panic and emerge to the surface, desperate for air. The wounds were soon clean and after a couple of injections, both goose and gander had a much more favourable prognosis. As I helped carry them to the car, the gander, whose lidless box I was carrying, made a bid for freedom. Luckily I managed to grab him, but as the consequences of a successful escape ran through my mind, the words of a Mr Men book from my childhood appeared: "There's a goose loose in the lane!"

Tom's DA

Tom had been busy with his usual farming jobs, but as the day progressed, he had become increasingly worried about one of his cows. She was off her food and off her milk. By six o'clock she was looking really poorly, so he decided to call the vet.

Evening surgery had just finished, so I grabbed what extra equipment I thought I might need- not just for Tom's cow, but for the rest of the night ahead as well. It is impossible to predict what a night on call might bring, so it is best to be prepared.

The signs that Tom reported over the phone sounded serious but it was hard to tell what the problem might be. All poorly cows go off their food and, quite quickly, look very sick. However, the fact that Tom was sufficiently worried to call me out in the evening was evidence enough that she was in a bad way.

And in a bad way she certainly was. The poor cow looked sick even from the far end of the collecting yard, where I parked my car. Her ears were droopy and so was her demeanour.

I greeted Tom, who looked tired and worried- it had been a long day and one that was far from over. The three most important questions to ask to a dairy farmer about a sick cow (vet students take note) are: When did she calve? How much milk did she give this morning? Did she eat her cake? This is not some Marie Antoinette-type interrogation, but a reference to whether the cow ate her breakfast (yes, cows eats cake for breakfast!)

Armed with this information, alongside a thermometer, a stethoscope and a lubricated rectal glove, a large animal vet can usually work out, with some confidence, what is wrong with a bovine patient. In a world crammed full of technology, it is a pleasant experience to diagnose an illness using a clinical history and a stethoscope. And it wasn't long before I'd made my diagnosis. This cow had calved just a couple weeks ago, she had not eaten her cake for breakfast, she'd been fine after calving but her milk had dropped off over the last couple of days. Her temperature was normal, but it was my stethoscope that gave me the answer. I placed it on her left flank to listen for rumen noises- there were barely any. I moved it lower down and flicked her muscular flank with my index finger, listening intently for the noise that would confirm my suspicion. Sure enough, there was a classic pinging noise, just like the noise you would get if you flicked the side of a metal drum, half full of water.

"PING, PING, PING," went the cow's left flank, each time I flicked it. The cow had a left displaced abomasum. Everything fitted in and, if I'm honest, I thought that this was a possibility as soon as I'd asked those first three questions. An abomasum displaced to the left is a condition that can affect recently calved cows. The abomasum- the fourth stomach of the cow- gets stuck behind the rumen, during the abdominal upheaval that occurs during and after calving. It should sit on the right, in the lower part of the abdomen but, trapped in the wrong place, it fills with gas and makes the cow poorly. The trapped gas and stomach fluid is the cause of the ping.

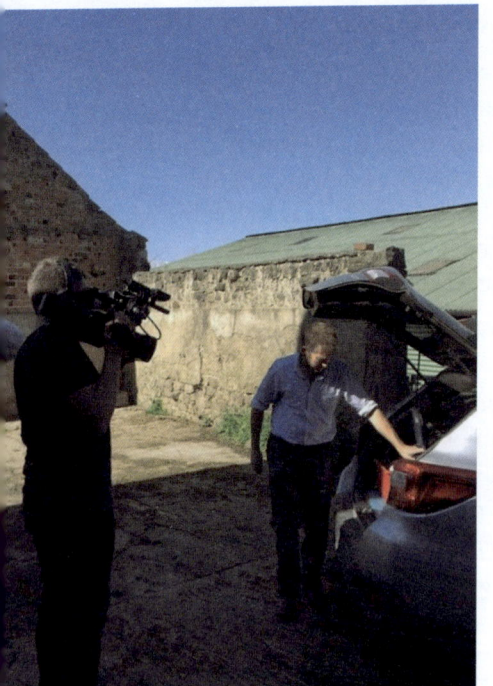

I explained the situation- and what I needed to do about it- to Tom. Experienced as he was, he hadn't seen this problem before so, before I reached for the local anaesthetic and my surgical kit, I set about talking through, in detail, what was about to unfold.

Arriving to see the sick cow. As ever, a camera pointing at me!

Tom's DA Continued

I talked through with Tom exactly what I was planning. His cow was poorly and, although a displaced abomasum operation is not an emergency – it's not like a twisted stomach in a dog, for example – she was pretty sick and it would have been foolish to delay the inevitable surgery, which would (we hoped) be life-saving.

We got her into Tom's excellent cattle crush, which had all manner of sophisticated mod-cons to allow perfect restraint of the cow and access to the surgical site. There are some farms that operate with antediluvian handling systems, rusting and fastened together with baler twine, which make handling cattle more challenging. This evening's operation would be under perfect conditions and both cow, vet and farmer would be safe from injury. Too many times I've risked bruised arms, damaged kneecaps, or worse, broken bones, because cattle have not been adequately restrained – but not this evening.

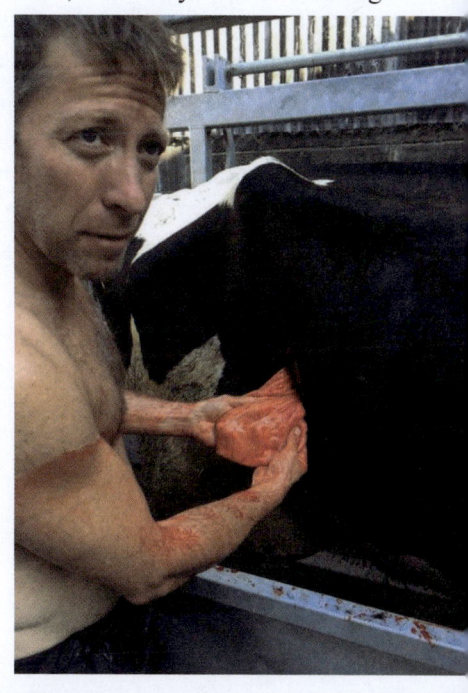

I have fixed many displaced abomasa, but today was an exciting day for me. Today was the day I tried a new surgical technique, which is always exciting. What needs to happen, to correct the condition, is for the abomasum to be repositioned from the left (abnormal) side, to the right (normal) side of her abdominal cavity. There are lots of ways of achieving this repositioning. One way, the one I've done most, is to use two vets, make two incisions in the cow – one on each side – and pass the abomasum from one vet to the other, literally with the arm of both vets inside the cow. It works well and is pretty fool-proof, but is time-consuming, two vets are needed (not great at 7.30 at night) and the cow has two incisions – one on each side. Another simple method, requiring just one vet but several helpers from the farm, is to role the cow onto her back, hold her legs still and make an incision under her abdomen. The displaced stomach floats into approximately the correct position when the cow is on her back. The surgical time is kept to a minimum, but this version requires lots of assistants and, whilst it is quick, cows do not really like being held upside down.

There are several other options, one of which I was about to embark upon this evening. It involved making a single incision in the right side of the cow, with her standing upright. I would reach across her abdomen, identify the displaced fourth stomach, squeeze it to allow gas to escape into the first part of the intestines, and then attempt to return it to the rightful place, just below my incision. In theory it was simpler, but required some skill and long arms, neither of which I had. Nonetheless, I knew it was the way forward as it is the method favoured by many cattle vets these days. Tom's Friesian would, therefore, be a guinea pig.

I took a deep breath and made my first cut, then tentatively explored the abdomen. Sure enough, a hugely distended abomasum was trapped on the left side of her abdomen. I felt a bit like someone embarking on a rescue attempt for a cave-diving accident, as I felt blindly at full arm's length. Tom was oblivious to the challenges I faced inside his cow's abdomen, which was maybe just as well.

Once I'd squeezed out some gas, the displaced organ was fairly easily manoeuvred into its correct position, and the fatty tissue adjacent to it was perfect to use to anchor it in place. Everyone felt happy with the evening's work, especially the cow, who walked off to join her herdmates, completely oblivious to what had been going on! It was early days, with much that could go wrong, but so far it was looking good!

Alpaca in the Practice

We have had a few unusual animals in the practice over the last couple of months. Dogs, cats and rabbits are the norm, but there have also been some ferrets and the odd hedgehog and, most recently, one or two alpacas. It always makes heads turn in the waiting room, or outside the surgery in New Row, Boroughbridge, when one of these elegant and leggy camelids walks down the road.

A little alpaca called "Hope" was born with a problem with one of her front legs. There was some pain and the leg deviated from the normal straight and narrow. I had tried some treatment, in the form of splints when she was smaller and injections as she got bigger. Neither seemed to help. Eventually, her owner Jackie and I decided we should take an X-ray of the leg. X-rays are always the next step when faced with a lameness that is not improving. The problem was I hadn't X-rayed many alpacas before. I knew what to do though. An alpaca's leg is, of course, comparable to that of similar creatures, so I could extrapolate my knowledge from other species. This is something veterinary surgeons do very frequently. We learnt *comparative* anatomy at vet school, which is exactly what the name suggests. It is impossible to learn every detail of every species, both in terms of anatomy, physiology and pathophysiology. So, instead, we learn from first principles, building up specific knowledge of the different groups of animals, and from there we can always work things out. This is one of the reasons that being a vet is so much fun and so challenging. The other thing which gave me confidence was that, while Hope had a bad leg, she also had a good leg, so the first job would be to take a radiograph of the good one. It would provide a perfect normal against which I could compare the bad leg.

But my biggest problem was actually working out the practicalities of the job. Lame horses (in most cases) can be X-rayed in situ, at the yard or stable. Modern X-ray machines can connect directly with a laptop and perfect, high-resolution images can be obtained instantly and horse-side. Instinctively, I started to think about loading up the X-ray kit to obtain the images at the farm. But Hope the alpaca was no bigger than a Labrador and I soon realised that it would probably be much simpler if I arranged for her to come to the practice.

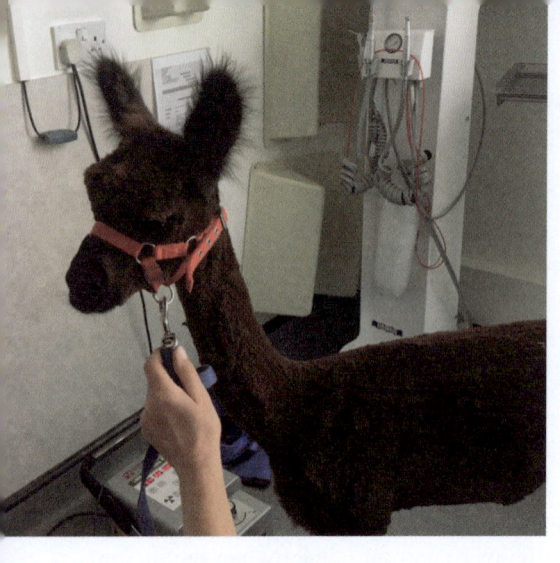

The next task was to rearrange the system. Dogs and cats are, by necessity, sedated and X-rayed lying on the X-ray table. They need to be motionless to get a good image. They also need to be in very specific positions, so the beams go through at the correct angle, highlighting exactly the correct bit to make a diagnosis. The X-ray beams go vertically downwards from a generator head above the patient and make the image on the screen underneath.

In Hope's case, I didn't really want to lie her on her side, as she was likely to struggle, so I decided to take the pictures using a horizontal beam, in the same way as we would in a horse. In this way, I managed to get perfect X-rays of the affected leg and also the good leg for comparison. Stage one completed!

Then I just had to work out the cause of the problem with her leg! I peered at the X-rays. Luckily, it was very clear: a classic case of an infection at the growth plate. No wonder she was lame and the leg deformed! I'd made a diagnosis. All that remained was for me to get Hope started on some treatment.

Another Alpaca in the Practice

"Hope" the lame alpaca was doing incredibly well. I had called Jackie, her owner, after about a week of treatment and the progress she reported was quicker and more complete than even an optimistic vet like me could have hoped for (yes, the pun had become very repetitive!).

It wasn't long before another alpaca visited the surgery. This one was much smaller. She was a week-old cria called Ivory, whose mum had been short of milk. This meant that the baby had not received sufficient colostrum – the first, nutrient-packed milk, which is full of protective antibodies. Without this protective elixir, many animals are susceptible to life-threatening infections as the immune system is so compromised.

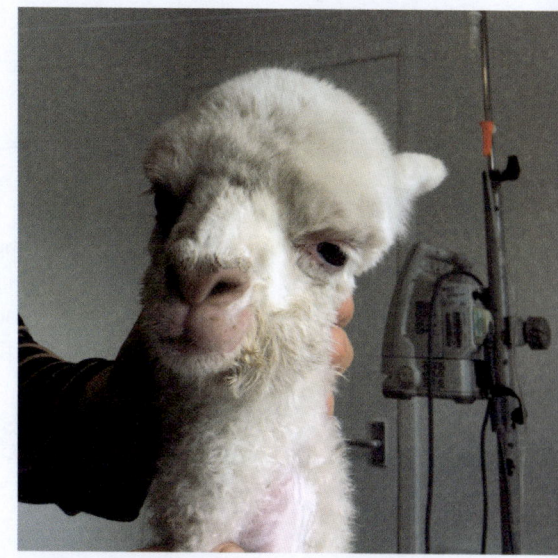

There is a solution to this problem, but it needs some prior planning. As the army say, "prior planning prevents poor performance" and so we had prepared, some time ago, by collecting bags of plasma, from healthy adult alpacas. The system is fiddly and involves the Pet Blood Bank, which offers a great service for handling blood donations in dogs and cats, allowing blood to be readily available if a pet needs a blood transfusion. They have adapted their services so that alpacas can benefit, too. I had collected about ten bags of blood, weighed and labelled each one and packaged them up in an insulated box. An ambulance-type van collected the box of blood and whisked it away to the lab, and a week later I had a supply of frozen plasma, ready for action in case of just the problem that faced Ivory.

We defrosted one of the frozen bags according to the instructions and Ivory arrived for her transfusion. The consulting room had been transformed into an emergency room and there was a tangible sense of excitement for everyone involved. I had done transfusions many times before, but for the owner and the nurses (and, of course, the camera crew), this was a first. The plasma bag was hung up and the drip line connected. I clipped fleece from Ivory's neck and prepped it thoroughly with scrub and surgical spirit, before taking a deep breath and placing the catheter. It can be difficult to put an intravenous cannula in a baby cria. Their skin is thick and the vein is small, although the process is easier once the thick fleece is removed.

The catheter slipped in easily and I applied some tissue glue to keep it in place. In the past, we used to place sutures to keep a catheter in the jugular vein of a horse or large animal (we use the front leg of a dog or cat), but nowadays, modern tissue glue – very much like superglue – works a treat. I hooked up the antibody-rich bag of fluid and watched it drip in slowly. Everyone crossed fingers that no abnormal reaction would occur. This is always a possibility and swelling of the face and other nasty things can happen if there is any type of transfusion reaction. I trickled the liquid in slowly at first, then more quickly as Ivory appeared to be coping very well. The tension in the room lifted as it became clear that everything was going to plan.

Within just a few minutes, all the new plasma was coursing through Ivory's veins. The boost to her immunity would cover the gap while her own immune system was inadequate. Meanwhile, for everyone watching and helping, there was also a boost. It wasn't additional plasma that had caused it, but the satisfaction of doing something new and life-saving. It had been a good morning's work and I hoped the outcome would be as successful as that of the previous alpaca in the practice!

Stanley and His Semen

Autumn is the time of year when sheep are ready to mate. Their oestrus activity is triggered by the shorter days and, given that the gestation length is just over five months, this means that lambs are born in the spring, when warmth is returning to the land and energising green grass is bursting into life in the sunny pastures. Nature is clever like that. Technically, therefore, preparation for lambing time has already started.

Tups have been purchased over the summer, if new genetic diversity is required on the farm. Existing tups are being preened so they are in good health for the busiest time of their year – extra food is offered and feet are trimmed to prevent lameness. Some tups need to be tested to confirm their fertility. It is frustrating and inefficient if a male is not firing on all cylinders, and can have big repercussions when spring arrives.

Stanley was one such tup and he was patiently waiting for me one afternoon recently, penned up in an old Yorkshire stone barn. Modern technology was about to meet old-fashioned and traditional, as I unloaded my equipment from the car. First though, I carried out a physical examination of the sturdy sheep. I palpated each testicle and measured their circumference. "The consistency of ripe tomatoes" was the aide-memoire instilled into us as vet students, to describe the ideal consistency of a healthy testicle. Happily, Stanley had a couple of beefsteaks sitting snugly in his scrotum. Their circumference went right past the mark I had made on my tape. It was easier to have an indelible mark than to remember an absolute figure: was it 32 or 34 centimetres? I always had to look it up!

Then it was time to reach for my kit. I needed a plug for my microscope. I also needed warm, glass slides, a flask containing water at exactly 37 degrees and, crucially, the electro-ejaculator. This device allows a sample of semen to be collected in a simple and relatively unobtrusive manner. I got everything ready, including

Stanley. The farmer held his head so he didn't move at the wrong moment. I lubricated the probe and inserted it up Stanley's bottom. Moments later [I won't bore you with the absolute details] I had a small sample of semen, collected in a plastic bag, nestling in the water bath to ensure it stayed at the correct temperature.

The next bit was the part I liked best. I loaded up a pipette and applied a small drop to the warmed glass slide, then peered down the microscope to see what was going on. This is very exciting. One minute I am looking at an actual animal, strong, stocky and healthy, the next, I am staring at cells, the building blocks of new life, measured in microns rather than kilograms. I love being able to make an assessment of a fully-grown animal and also to assess its cells at a microscopic level.

Stanley's semen had the appearance of swirling smoke from a bonfire made of autumnal leaves, which confirmed that everything was good. There is no requirement for an absolute sperm count, but rather an assessment of morphology and motility. If too many sperms are dead or defective, this swirling motion doesn't exist and the sample appears static. It is a subjective test that requires knowledge and experience. Stanley's sample showed that he had excellent semen quality. I gave the thumbs up to his owner. He was fully active and ready to go. Unperturbed by the whole process, he ambled out to grass. He would have a busy time in the coming weeks, but for now he was totally unaware of the responsibilities resting on his testicles.

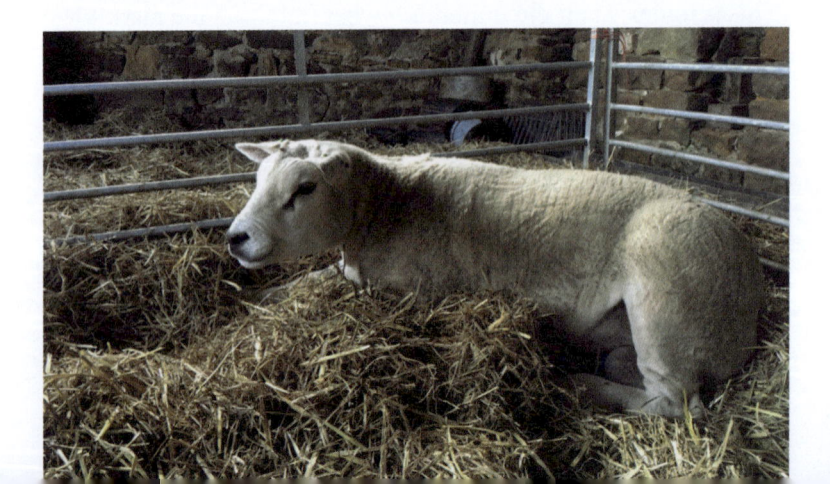

Pregnant but Broken

One of my colleagues had a dilemma. She had seen an emergency case over the weekend – a young cat called Smokey, with a broken leg. This wasn't the dilemma – the broken bone clearly needed to be fixed and the X-rays showed that this would be a simple enough job. Cats' legs are often relatively easy to repair. The bones are quite straight and heal quickly, and cats tend to tolerate injuries well, without feeling sorry for themselves. There are occasions when we happen to treat stray or feral cats, who have suffered car accidents earlier in their life and have horribly deformed legs, where fractures have healed naturally, without any veterinary intervention. Whilst this is not a good thing, it serves to highlight the point that cats have an amazing knack of repairing themselves.

This particular fracture would not be one that would repair properly without intervention, though. The front leg hung limp and floppy. The complicating factor was that the young cat was pregnant, so there was much more at stake than just repairing a floppy leg. But, there was no way we could postpone surgery until after the kittens had been born – the quicker a fractured bone is stabilised, the quicker the pain is alleviated. Stability is the best painkiller for a broken bone, whether this takes the form of an emergency supporting bandage, a splint, a cast or a repair with internal metalwork. We needed to minimise any anaesthetic risk to the unborn kittens, so I made my plan, organised myself and got everything ready to make sure the surgery went smoothly. I needed to be quick, efficient and careful.

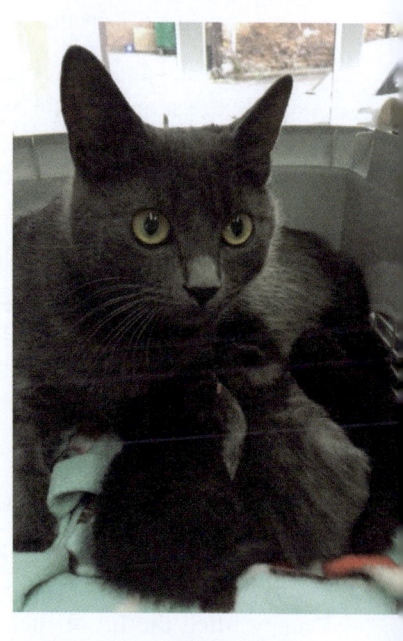

I am not a brilliant orthopaedic surgeon – I'm certainly no *Super Vet*, and my efforts with drills and screwdrivers around the house are functional rather than accomplished (and Anne always looks worried when I reach for the tool box), but I relish the challenge of restoring function to a broken leg. I set about the task with vigour, explaining as I went along what I was doing and why I was doing it, to our vet student and anyone else who was interested. The fractured ends came together well and normal rigidity was quickly restored. I took a final X-ray to confirm everything was back in line, and then sutured the muscle layers and skin, happy with the outcome. I felt confident the bones would heal, but we still had to cross our fingers for the baby kittens.

Once we had applied a bandage, to protect the suture line and add some extra support, little Smokey was ready to go home. She would need a few bandage changes over the next few weeks, as well as suture removal, so I scheduled some follow-up appointments.

Everything went well. Smokey was soon free of her stitches and then her bandages and her pregnancy seemed to be progressing according to plan. So, when her name appeared on the appointment list a few weeks later, I was worried that something had gone wrong. Had the pin moved? Was it encroaching on the adjacent joints? Was Smokey lame again? Had some infection crept into the surgical site?

I called Smokey and her owners into the consulting room.

"Is everything alright?" I asked, cautiously.

"Everything is absolutely fine," nodded her owners. "She's doing very well. Her leg has healed a treat, but we've brought her back." They lifted the lid off her plastic cat-carrier, and continued, "We thought you'd like to see these!"

Inside the box was Smokey, sound and solid of leg, sitting proudly next to a pile of little, fluffy kittens. It was another happy day in the clinic!

Milk Fever

I had an urgent call last Friday night. Richard, the farmer, had gone to check on a bunch of cows and heifers, grazing away from the farm. They were making the most of late-season grass. One of the cows was lying on her side when he arrived. The sight of a farmer in his pickup usually brings cattle running, anticipating an extra bag of food. This poor cow though, couldn't stand up, so Richard called me straightaway, concerned about the possibility of milk fever, or worse the dreaded staggers!

Milk fever is not some sort of illness brought about by an intolerance to lactose, but a deficiency in the blood calcium levels, usually seen in older cows, soon after calving, as the calcium that usually is in the blood is diverted to the udder to make milk. It results in muscle weakness and affected animals cannot stand up. If it's not addressed, it is very serious and the cow can die.

Staggers is altogether more dramatic and is the result of a drop in blood magnesium. The condition progresses very quickly, with cows shaking and trembling their way to a rapid death. Both conditions start off with a cow lying on its side, and Richard was worried about staggers. Hence his urgent call for my help.

"She's not at the farm, though," he added just before I rang off. "Meet me at the farm and you can follow me there. It's hard to explain exactly where the field is."

I arrived at his farm just as dusk was descending and duly followed the rickety old pickup truck as it wound along the quiet lanes, overhung with hedges. Finally, Richard pulled into a layby and got out.

"You might want to get a lift with me from here," he offered. "It's a bit rutty and bumpy and it might damage the underneath of your car."

Usually, I relish the chance to test the off-road capabilities of my

Subaru and I love treating cattle *al fresco*. I also prefer to have all my equipment to hand, in my car boot, but I deferred to his greater knowledge of the field and collected everything I thought I might need: bottles of calcium and magnesium – to treat either or both conditions – thermometer, stethoscope, rectal glove and lubricant. I shoved a halter into my pocket and grabbed some syringes, some smaller bottles of medicine and some needles. I'd need the big, wide-bored ones to allow the calcium or magnesium solutions to run in quickly through the rubber flutter valve – a special tube to attach directly to the mouth of the mineral bottle. The needles were different to those I usually used. Supply problems meant they were a different colour, but as long as they were wide, it didn't matter who made them. I tucked a handful into the chest pocket of my shirt.

The cow was easy to catch, seeing as she couldn't stand. She didn't relish the idea of being restrained, though. She obviously thought that, since this was a field, cattle should be left to roam freely and she flung her head around to avoid examination. Her calf peered at us from afar and, even though it was now dark, she had a good view of the action under the headlights of Richard's vehicle.

Once I had managed to examine her, I decided that calcium was the cure. I removed the lid from a bottle and attached my rubber valve in readiness to run the life-saving elixir into her jugular vein. Now for the needle. I pulled off the cap, only to discover, to my dismay, that it was hopelessly too narrow! As I watched the calcium trickle in at a fraction of the usual speed, I knew we were in for a long night!

Enzo and His Bad Eye

Poor Enzo had the shortest consultation ever. The little French bulldog puppy didn't even make it as far as my consulting room, as I whisked him away from his distraught owner and ran with him directly into theatre.

"Reception will sort you out with a consent form," I shouted over my shoulder. "And I'll give you a ring when I'm done."

I felt bad and I felt a bit rude. I usually try to spend some time explaining to an owner the various options for treatment and possible complications, even in an emergency, but in Enzo's case there was no time and actually no need for such a conversation. Another dog had attacked the little pup, who was just a few months old. His left eyeball had prolapsed – that is, it had popped out of its socket. So, there was little need for discussion and a lot of need for action.

Even though it looks like something from a joke shop, a prolapsed globe is a genuine veterinary emergency and needs immediate attention. Firstly, it is obviously very painful. The quicker it can be replaced, the sooner the pain subsides. Secondly, the longer the eye is out, bulging and swollen, with haemorrhage behind it and stretching of the optic nerve, the lower the chance of saving the eye. So, I felt justified in being a bit rude. Enzo was under anaesthetic within minutes of entering the building. It was maybe the shortest wait of all time!

As his anaesthetic stabilised, I ran through in my head what I needed to do. It is a horrible sight, and mercifully rather rare.

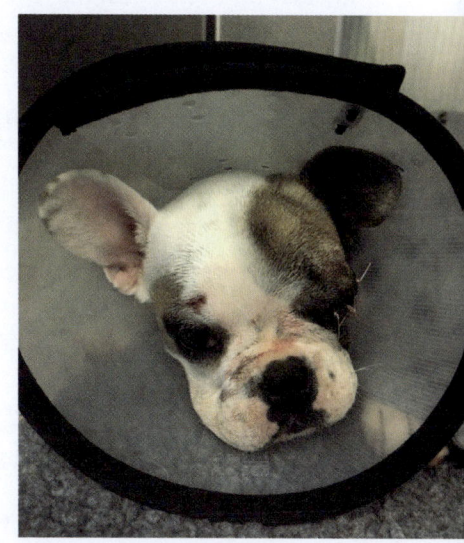

Cat and dog breeds with bulging eyes (and therefore shallow eye sockets) are more at risk, but any traumatic injury to the face or head can result in this horrendous condition.

Once Enzo was asleep, I made an incision at the lateral corner of his eye, where the upper and lower lids met. This is called a *lateral canthotomy*, which sounds very technical, but is actually just a small cut with a scalpel to create a bigger hole through which to replace the globe. The next job was to place sutures in the eyelids, to allow them to be pulled upwards over the prolapsed eye. Then I applied gentle but firm and constant pressure to the globe. The textbooks call this part *retropulsion of the globe*, which basically just means "pushing it back in".

After several minutes of retropulsion of the globe, I felt happy that it was back in its normal position so fastened the sutures together, to keep it in place. Enzo was quickly round from his anaesthetic and sitting up, plastic cone on head, as if nothing had happened.

I made the call to his owner, who I felt sure would be waiting anxiously, brandy in hand, by the phone.

"Hi, it's Julian here, from the vet's. Just an update about Enzo. He's absolutely fine and ready to go home whenever is convenient. I'm fairly hopeful we have saved his eye. I must apologise for being so rude before. I felt awful that I just grabbed him from you without any discussion . . ." I tried to explain and apologise at the same time.

When he was ready to go, I carried him out in just the same way he had come in, an hour earlier. Enzo wagged his stumpy tail with vigour. It's amazing how resilient dogs are. There's no time for feeling sorry for yourself when you're a dog.

His owner was altogether happier too. As I carried Enzo to the car, there were more tears, but this time they were tears of relief!

Podcast

"Guess what I'm doing next Friday?" I asked my kids one evening this week, after school. Both Jack and Archie shrugged. It could have been anything and neither of my boys is surprised by my antics nowadays. Over the last few years I have done many things that I could never have expected, so it really was impossible for them to guess. They are also teenagers, so shrugging is a thing.

"I'm headlining a festival," I said, grinning. They had both been to Leeds Festival, during the summer, where they had seen the likes of Bastille and the Foo Fighters, who were also headline acts. We all knew that *my* gig would not be very similar.

Some weeks ago, I received an email from my neighbour and friend, Kate Fox. Kate is a very funny and very talented performance poet – a modern version of Pam Ayres (maybe). Over the last few years, we have done a series of evening events called *An evening with Julian Norton*, where we both sit on stage and have a conversation, talking about all sorts of things. It started small and local, but we have been as far as Lancaster, Hull and Scunthorpe! We have actually filled venues and, yes, people do pay to come and listen to us! We've hosted audiences of nearly five hundred people! To my never-ending astonishment, they seem to be fairly popular. Kate is very funny and accustomed to being on stage and makes it very easy for me. She has her own successful series of "gigs" (the most recent is *Where There's Muck There's Bras*) and she has regularly presented Radio 4's *Pick of the Week*. Since we are neighbours, transport is also simple.

On the way home from once such evening, conversation turned to the topic of podcasts. Neither of us knew very much about them, although we both knew they were popular. I have several friends who evangelise about these bite-sized audio logs, so we decided to have a go at making one, by recording our next event. Kate had experience of live recording, having been a radio journalist in a previous life (she recounts her breakthrough story was a scoop on the discovery of a frog in a bag of supermarket salad), so she could make a rough-cut edit of our performance.

At Darlington's Hullabaloo theatre, where episode one was recorded (live!), we canvassed the audience for suggestions for a suitable title for said podcast. The verdict, carried unanimously, was that the title should be *The Naked Vet*. This seemed apt, partly because of the recent discussions about the suitability of vets removing their shirts to perform surgery on cows. The fact that the whole show would be in audio form would save the audience any disappointment and save me from any feelings of objectification. The title has apparently stuck (although one member of the audience suggested a better name might be *The Naked Fox*. Neither Kate nor I thought this would really work).

So, on the evening of Friday 22 November, at Rural Arts in Thirsk, Kate and I will be headlining a festival of podcasts. The event is the inaugural event of the PODCAST SOCIAL CLUB, organised by the hugely popular and successful Deer Shed Festival. There are several other, established and already popular podcasts being recorded over this exciting weekend (notably one called "Desert Island Dicks", which asks which items or characters would make life on a desert island a living hell!).

For me, it's another step into the unknown! Let's hope it works!

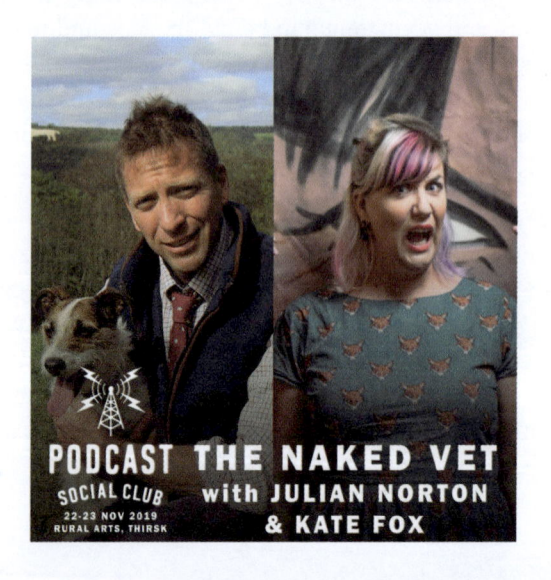

Confusacat

I saw a cat called Pipkin this week. It was a follow-up from his first consultation exactly two weeks before.

"There's something not right with him," explained his owner on that occasion. "He's sitting in odd places, staring at the wall, getting up in the night and making odd noises. It's as if he's become confused!" It sounded like an episode from *Monty Python's Flying Circus*!

I asked all the usual questions about his eating, drinking and so on. How long had this been going on for? Were there any identifiable trigger factors? I was searching carefully for clues, even before I had reached for my stethoscope, thermometer or blood sampling equipment. The answers can often be hinted at before any actual diagnostic tests are done.

The sixteen-year-old's appetite was reduced. He still ate, but with less enthusiasm, and, "Yes," his owner confirmed, "he is drinking more than before, now you come to mention it."

And yes, these things did all start at the same time. I was making progress and already had enough information to start working out a plan. I checked Pipkin all over, from head to tail. The whites of his eyes were white and not jaundiced yellow; his gums were pink and not pale and his teeth, on which I commented, were remarkably clean for a sixteen-year-old. There was no soreness of the gums and no mouth pain. Moving down his neck, his lymph nodes and thyroid glands were normal, as were his heart rate, chest cavity, lungs and trachea. These were all good things, but not helping me.

I put down my stethoscope and started

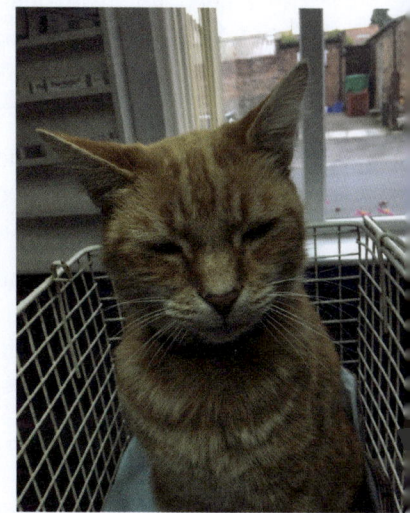

palpating Pipkin's abdomen. There are lots of structures in an abdomen. Luckily for a vet, cats have relaxed abdominal muscles and their abdominal cavity is relatively small, so it is quite easy to feel around.

I probed under Pipkin's spine and ran my fingers over each kidney. They were both knobbly and slightly swollen. Prodding them more firmly was definitely sore. Whilst this was not very nice for the cat, it was *very* helpful for the vet, looking for the answer to explain his clinical signs. Kidneys should not be bumpy, swollen or painful. If they are any of these things, then there is usually a problem with them – either an infection (something called pyelonephritis, which is fairly common in cats), or cancer (a bad thing).

Everything else in the abdomen seemed to be normal. I reached for my thermometer to take Pipkin's temperature. I needed one final piece of evidence to complete my diagnosis, which was duly provided by the thermometer reading of one hundred and three degrees.

"I think Pipkin has a kidney infection," I announced, before explaining my rationale. Bizarrely, a bit like in old people, kidney infections in cats can cause delirium. I do not know why, and I've never seen it written down in a book, but I've seen it in numerous cats and dogs over the years. An elderly Border Terrier called Cookie, was the last animal I saw with this problem, just a few weeks ago.

I explained my plan, which was to inject an antibiotic whose activity lasted for two weeks. This was ideal, because not only did this particular drug work well for kidney infections, but it meant confused Pipkin didn't need to be persuaded to take tablets.

So, when I saw Pipkin and his owner exactly two weeks later, I was excited to see whether I had made the correct diagnosis and whether the cat was less confused.

"It's quite amazing, Julian! He's completely back to normal!" effused his owner, very much relieved to have her cat back to his old self. I added Pipkin to my list of patients confounding the textbooks!

Goldfish, Open Mouth and Fake News

The final patient of the day came as a surprise to both of us. I was surprised because I don't see many goldfish and the patient . . . well, he looked absolutely horrified. This was because the poor goldfish, swimming around in its see-through container, appeared to be unable to close his mouth. He resembled the "surprised" emoji, wide-eyed and round-mouthed. Fish do not usually have the ability to change their facial expression. I learnt this at vet school, during my studies in embryology. The muscles that are used to provide facial expression in mammals form part of the gills in fish, where their role is simply to open and close to allow oxygen to diffuse from the water to the fish. It is a fascinating example of both comparative anatomy and of evolution and provides the explanation for the inability of fish to smile or frown.

But surprised as this fish looked, there was clearly a serious problem with his health, even though he appeared to be swimming normally. It is impossible to examine a goldfish with thoroughness. They live in water and should not be handled if possible, for fear of damaging their protective slimy layer. I would have to rely on textbooks and internet searches for the answer.

"I'm not sure there's much you'll be able to do for him," offered his owner.

Obviously she too realised that there were limited examination and treatment options. I acknowledged my shortcomings in this regard, confirming I was not a fish vet.

"I think it might be to do with his water," I suggested. "When was it last changed? Can you check the ammonia levels?"

This pretty much exhausted my limited knowledge, but I felt sure it was the most likely reason for the problem. Goldfish are very sensitive to elevated levels of ammonia and their water needs to be changed regularly, but only up to one third of its volume at a time. It is also crucial to use dechlorinated water.

I stared at the fish, trying to see if anything was stuck in his mouth – some pebbles or something from his tank. It seemed unlikely, but worth checking. The open mouth seemed free of obstruction.

For thoroughness, I sought the help of my textbooks, which confirmed the ammonia issue as the most likely cause. I then turned to the internet, where I thought a veterinary discussion forum might shed some more light on the problem. A quick search led me to a site that sounded ideal. It had the words "goldfish" and "emergencies" and ".com" in its title. I clicked on it, immediately finding lots of startled-looking goldfish, open-mouthed like the one in front of me. I was hopeful of more accurate information and scrolled further down the page. Another possible diagnosis appeared before my eyes, one that I had not even considered – TETANUS! I read on, intrigued. It described goldfish and koi carp as particularly at risk, because they were "bottom feeders". The thought of this habit made me recoil, until I realised it referred to the bottom of the tank or pond. The website went on further, dispelling the cause of *lockjaw*, the other name for tetanus, from rusty nails as "just a rumour". Constipation, it said, rather than rusty nails, in fish could lead to this nasty disease. By now I was concerned at the accuracy of the information. A few short sentences later, as it described tetanus as a "deadly virus" [it is, in fact, a disease caused by the toxin of the bacterium Clostridium Tetani – definitely NOT a virus], I had concluded that this emergency website for goldfish was full of fake news.

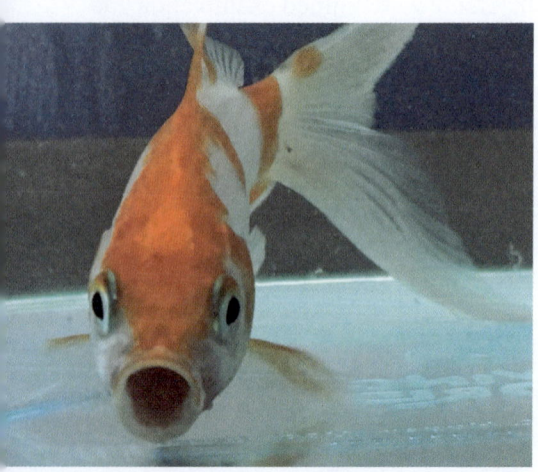

I decided to make my diagnosis and treatment plan without its help: he definitely needed new water!

Tiny Tim and Painful Prostates

It had been a busy morning, rather strangely, full of dogs with problematic or painful prostates. For some reason, there are a lot of entire (i.e. not castrated) dogs around Boroughbridge. I don't know why – maybe it reflects the rural nature of the area, or the fact that the dogs are spread more thinly and are therefore less likely to be affected by problems connected with testosterone. My first dog, a faithful and cuddly Border terrier, was castrated when he was about two years old. The increasing frequency with which he growled and threatened other male dogs on the pavements of Sowerby was becoming awkward. He thought it was his patch and his patch alone. The final straw came when he decided to pick a fight with a neighbour's dog while we stood chatting. Anne, my wife and fellow vet, and I took him straight to the practice and castrated him post-haste. It cured his tendencies for dominance in the village immediately.

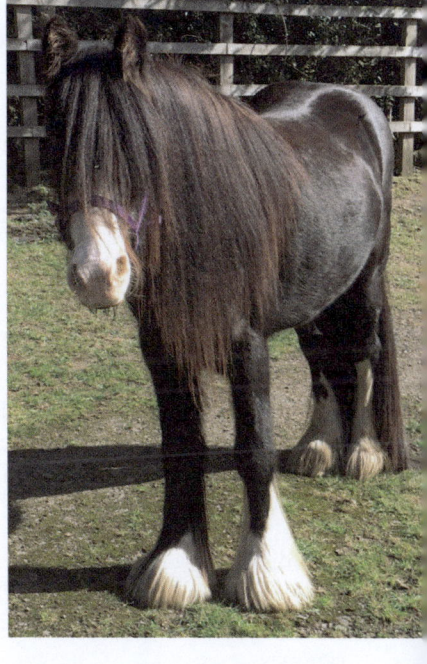

But, for the dog population of Boroughbridge, more testicles also equals more prostatic disease (the prostates of castrated males become smaller, inert and problem-free) and on this morning I had inserted my finger and palpated the firm, enlarged and irregular glands of a sedated Doberman and several Labradors. I'd taken X-rays and done ultrasound scans and even inserted a narrow needle to extract cells from two of these enlarged glands, in an attempt to find the cause of the problem. It's interesting stuff and I hoped the lab would provide me with a diagnosis in both cases.

So, after a busy morning in a darkened room with X-rays and ultrasounds, I was pleased to be heading out after lunch, into the sunshine. The first job was easy – a pony to vaccinate – but I wondered why the owner had specifically requested me. I looked up the notes to check which vaccine was needed and confirm the address. I'd been there a year ago to do the same job, although I had little recollection of the visit and couldn't remember the yard or the directions, let alone the animal. I set off, hopeful that it would come flooding back once I got nearby.

It didn't at first (I got lost twice) and the phone number I'd written down was incorrect, so I was glad when my memory finally kicked back into action to help me find the right lane. Once I pulled into the yard, I recognised the pony immediately. It was Tiny Tim! I'd met him a year ago, shortly after he'd arrived on the yard as a rescue, found unwanted on Facebook.

"I saw him on the computer, read his sad story and I just had to help," recalled his owner, recounting the time she'd first seen his picture online. I remembered his story. I had checked his teeth to try to confirm his age – I'd judged him to be about five – and examined him all over. The poor lad, not unlike his namesake in *A Christmas Carol*, was not a picture of health. However, I was hopeful that plenty of love, affection and food would put Tiny Tim back on track.

He did look a picture of health today though, his shiny coat and luxurious mane reflecting in the early winter sun. I patted his neck and rubbed his muzzle, keeping my vaccine in my pocket, out of sight.

"I asked for you to come today," explained his owner, "because I thought you'd like to see how handsome he's become in just a year!"

I had to agree. I also had to agree that, particularly on this day, ponies were definitely preferable to prostates!

Back to Back

Archie came in to see us with a new problem. The elderly terrier had been struggling with a nasal discharge for some months, which we had more or less under control. Nasal disease can be complicated, both to get a diagnosis and to treat. It is hard to take representative samples up a nose, especially as the important bits are actually quite a long way in. Unless it's a pug or similar, a dog's nose is much longer than a human's. It is also extremely difficult to operate on. Medication is usually the mainstay of treatment, and this was the case with Archie.

His recent problem, however, was his back and not his nose. Pain and then neurological signs had developed quite quickly and our X-rays identified some very narrowed disc spaces between some of the bones of his spine. Under these circumstances, the discs – similar to rubber washers – get squeezed upwards and into the spinal canal, squashing the nerves of the spinal cord. Archie would need an MRI and possibly spinal surgery, both of which were outside our capabilities at Boroughbridge.

MRI machines work by a combination of massive, spinning magnets, protons and magic to make detailed images of the parts of the body that X-rays cannot reach. They came into veterinary use some time after I left vet school and I have never learnt about their workings, so I presume magic is a key ingredient to their success.

We sent Archie to a brand-new, state-of-the-art, specialist referral centre, Swift Referrals, happily very nearby in Thorpe Arch. This offered Archie the best chance of his problem being identified and fixed. By the next day he was walking, happy and like a new dog. They had done a great job.

By coincidence, I too had been up close and personal with the inside of an MRI machine. I'd been warned it was an unpleasant experience, claustrophobic and noisy, but in reality, lying on my back, eyes closed for twenty minutes, with no phone ringing and nobody asking me to calve a cow, blood-sample their cat or fix their hamster, was quite relaxing. I was hoping my diagnosis was going to be as simple as Archie's.

I was handed a CD containing the vital information about my back, its health and ill-health, but the imagers wouldn't let me look at it at the hospital, and a normal laptop wouldn't show the images. No matter, by the end of the day, and I won't say how, I'd managed to view the slices of my spinal cord. I made all sorts of diagnoses – to me it looked very similar to Archie's back (although with fewer vertebrae. At first, when I'd heard the clinicians talking about my L5-S1 junction, I presumed *this* was the reason I was of only average height – I was missing two vertebrae! It turns out though that, while dogs have seven lumbar vertebrae, humans only have five!

Once I realised I didn't even know the basics, I stopped trying to self-diagnose. This was a job for people who knew what they were talking about. It was discombobulating to have a problematic backbone. It is literally and figuratively the thing that is crucial, strong and connecting. Apparently, with one metaphor too many, mine was also my Achilles heel. I should not have been surprised. Days spent stooped over a consulting table, being contorted at odd angles whilst taking blood samples from the underside of cows' tails, heaving heavy calves from the worst of positions and lifting the feet of implausibly heavy horses had obviously taken their toll. Add in miles of pounding the woods and trails of Yorkshire in my running shoes over the years and it was, in short, buggered. Like Archie, I'd be needing the help of a very specialist surgeon.

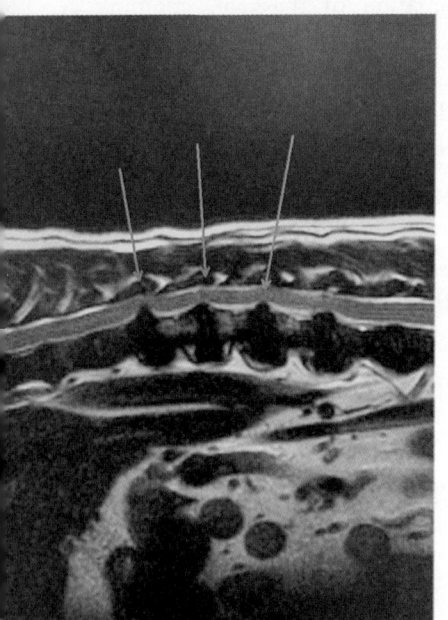

Image of Archie's spine.

Christmas at the Vet's

Christmas is upon us. For a vet during the festive season, it is very much a case of business as usual. Animals, whether a constipated cat, a wheezing Westie or a calving cow, do not know about Christmas. They do not know about bank holidays, nor about spending time with the family and enjoying delicious seasonal meals.

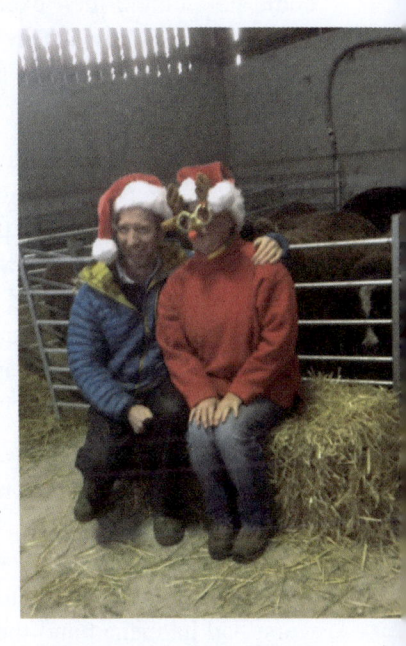

Time off over the festive period is shared out, but the general precedent is that vets with small children have first dibs at the rota. I remember one year being on call on Christmas Eve, but off duty on Christmas Day to allow my young kids to spend some time with their dad, unencumbered by a beeper and on-call responsibilities. It had been a busy night. Calving a cow at two a.m. was actually a wonderful experience. The farmer and his wife were embarrassed at calling the vet when it should have been Santa out delivering things, but a healthy calf and a happy cow was the earliest and best Christmas present they could have wished for. I had delivered countless of their lambs and calves over the years and it was a privilege to be the first to wish two of my farming friends a happy Christmas on that frosty night. It was just like a nativity scene – cows were literally eating from a manger and lowing softly. Sadly, I don't think the calf was christened Jesus. I suppose that would have been wrong. I went back to bed briefly, but then, like children all over the world, I rose early. I had inpatients to check – catheters to flush, bladders to empty. I also had a turkey to cook. I reckoned that it would take an hour or so, and I rose at four thirty, intending to be back before six so I could watch our young kids open their presents. The proper magic of Christmas.

My plan failed. The catheters and bladders took a bit longer than expected and my kids got up earlier than I expected. They were as excited as you'd imagine – Father Christmas had been in the night and filled their stockings. On finding my car once again not in the drive, they presumed I was tied up with work (I was). They could not contain their excitement. I returned home, shortly after six thirty on Christmas Day morning, to find Anne half asleep, two overexcited kids and a big pile of screwed-up wrapping paper. I'd missed it all!

On my first ever Christmas on call, I went to see an old man who had an elderly terrier. Both the owner, whose name was Mr Moss, and his canine companion, had the same problem – severe emphysema. We visited him regularly, when the dog's lung function dipped to a serious level. The steroid injections we gave seemed to provide relief for a few months, but apparently the drugs had worn off at eleven o'clock on Christmas Day morning. The terrier's breathing was bad and my beeper went off with a call to his house.

Because I'd visited the house several times before, I knew Mr Moss and his dog lived alone. The wheezing dog was all the company he had on Christmas Day. I checked my emergency box. It was full of all I would need – stethoscope, syringes, drugs, and even the equipment necessary to administer the final injection if the worst had happened and the terrier's lungs had deteriorated to an impossible state of health (thankfully, that wasn't the case). But as I headed out of my front door, I had a thought. I had forgotten some essential kit. I went back into the kitchen and grabbed a box of mince pies and a half-opened bottle of Merlot, which Mr Moss and I shared after I'd treated his dog. They were not conventional medicines, but those mince pies were the best treatment I'd dispensed all year!

Stories of New Year's Eve Past

New Year, for a vet, is very similar to Christmas. In most practices, it forms part of the "Christmas Rota", so you either work one or the other.

But being on call on New Year's Eve can be fun. A couple of years ago, I delivered a litter of pups at two in the morning, by caesarean section. I wished the owners a Happy New Year when they arrived at the practice; I wished Katy, my colleague whom I had to call in to assist me, a Happy New Year. Then we had the privilege of wishing a Happy New Year to each of six tiny puppies as they squeaked their first squeaks. Bringing new life into the world was a good start to the New Year! Much better than nursing a hangover, like much of the country.

Another year, I was called at a similar time of night, in the small hours. This time it was to a cow belonging to John, a farmer, who had just got home from a New Year's Eve party. Despite being somewhat the worse for wear, he had diligently set about checking his stock before going to bad. He'd spotted a cow that had just calved and called me immediately.

"Thank goodness, Julian," he slurred anxiously down the phone. "I've just got back from the pub and this cow has calved and she's pushed her calf bed out."

A "calf bed out" is the lay term for a prolapsed uterus. It is a serious problem and one that demands strenuous, messy exertion and some skill. I braced myself for a tough job on that freezing cold and crystal clear New Year's morning. When I arrived, I found John staggering around, sloshing water over the side of the bucket he was carrying, as he meandered across the dark farm yard, illuminated by the light of his mobile phone and a full bright moon. I parked, got my wellies on and left the car engine running and headlights on, to provide some much-needed extra light. He beckoned me over and I followed, avoiding muddy puddles of indeterminate depth. I did not want to fall into a deep one because, judging by the drunken phone call and John's wandering, I did not think he'd be able to help me out.

We met by the gate and peered into the yard of cattle. I hoped the patient would be easy to get hold of, but she was not even easy to identify, let alone catch.

"Which one is she, John?" I asked, peering into the darkness. "Oh, and Happy New Year!"

"And a very Happy New Year to you. It's the brown one," slurred the inebriated farmer, referring to the patient rather than the new year. It certainly wasn't going to be a brown year. "She's over there! Near the calf."

But when we climbed over the gate to try and catch the patient, it turned out she wasn't a patient at all.

"John, that's not a prolapsed uterus! It's just some cleansing. She's fine. I can go back to bed!" Cleansing is the remains of the placenta and is completely normal to see after a calf is born. What a relief!

But possibly the most memorable of all New Year's calls was to see a whole herd of cows. Overnight, the cows had enjoyed their own party and broken into the feed store, gorging themselves on cow-cake. The result was acidosis, the signs of which look very much like a person who is drunk. The sight that met me, around eight in the morning on New Year's Day, was very similar to the scene in towns, pubs and houses all over the country, as pretty much the whole herd staggered, drunk and disorderly around the farmyard.

I wonder what's in store for me this New Year?

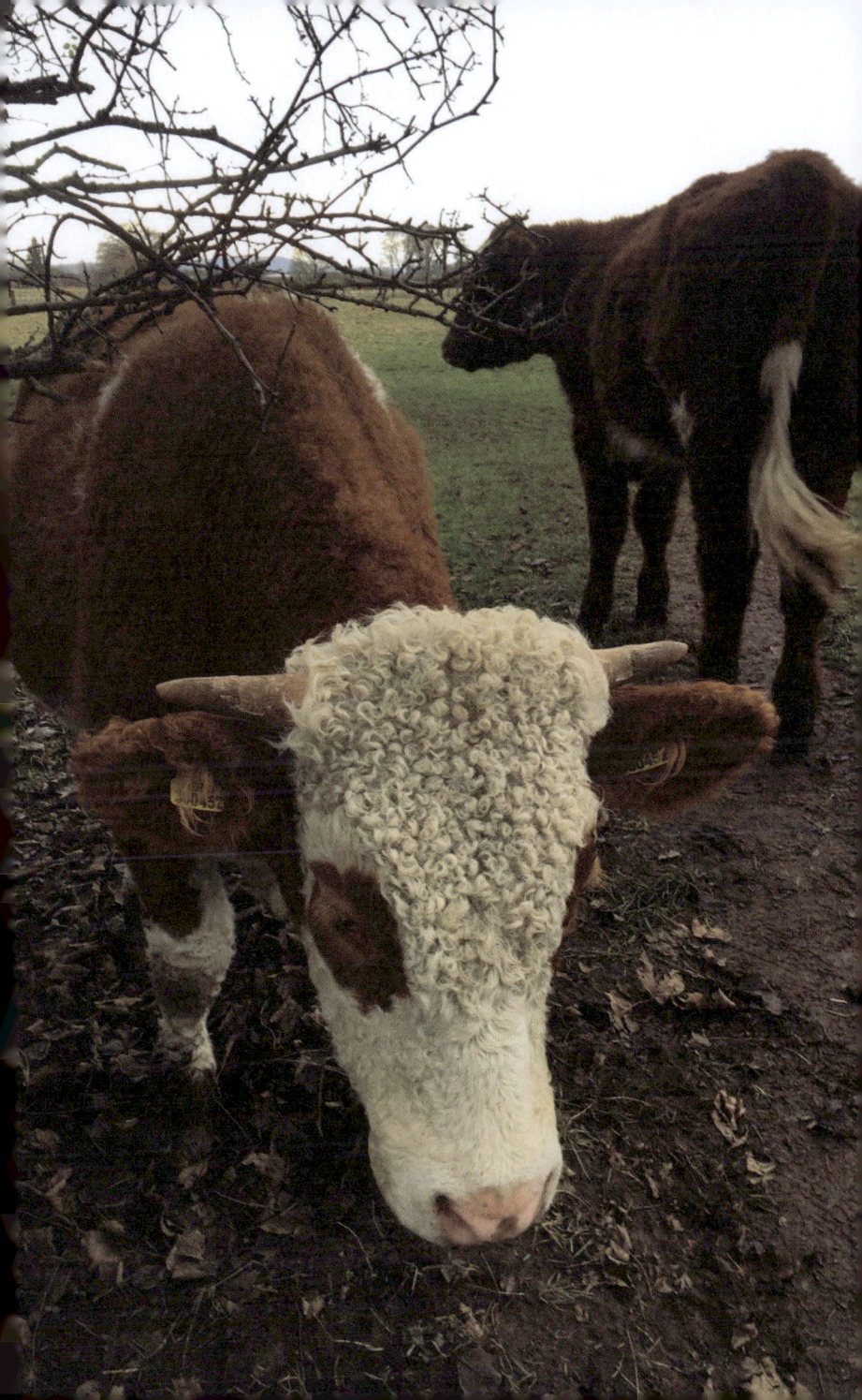

I've Got a Fleam

I've had a few interesting gifts from grateful clients over the years. The lamp, in the shape of a bulldog with a lampshade on top of its head, which is looking at me as I write this column, is probably the most memorable. It was a gift to remind me of a favourite patient called Elsie. One of my kids keeps asking,

"How long is that ridiculous lamp going to stay in the kitchen?"

"As long as it makes me smile," is my answer.

Elsie's double keeps putting a smile on my face and so remains supervising each mealtime in our house.

But I had another unusual gift recently. It came from the widow of Trevor, a neighbour of my parents, and it used to belong to her husband. When I was a child, I spent many a happy summer day at their house, learning about ferrets, whittling sticks with penknives and pointing air rifles at tin cans with their son, Jason. Trevor was very keen that this object was passed on to me.

It looked just like a beautifully crafted penknife, with a perfect bone handle and smoothly inset pins to keep the blades in place. But when I opened the blades, it became evident that it was not a penknife. The three blades did have a sharp edge, but curved and triangular with a pointy end and each of a different size. I had never seen anything like it and so some research was required.

Google came into its own. I typed in the manufacturer's name, which was inscribed on one of the blades, and straightaway the "images" section of said search engine gave me an answer. It was a *fleam*. A bit more investigation revealed that a fleam (also known as a flem, flew, flue or phleam) is (or more specifically, was) an instrument to puncture a blood vessel and thereby facilitate a procedure called "blood-letting". The blade of the appropriate size was placed over the jugular vein of a horse and hit with a stick. After the appropriate amount of blood was deemed to have drained out, the hole was stitched up with a pin and piece of hair from the horse's own tail!

Of course, in times of antiquity, before there was any scientific basis for therapeutic treatments, this was practised for pretty much any condition. Leeches were also used in people to suck out blood and badness. We now know that this is not helpful. There is just one condition called *polycythaemia*, in which the blood has too many red blood cells, where it might be, but it is rare. It seems highly unlikely that any patients – human or equine – in that bygone era would have been suffering from the one specific and rare condition that would have benefitted from this treatment. And yet it took until the late nineteenth century for the practice to disappear. Or so I thought.

I was recently perusing the first few chapters of the Herriot classic *If Only They Could Talk*. I read the passage where James arrives in Darrowby for a job interview. Mr Farnon, who had apparently forgotten about the interview, is hopelessly late but eventually appears and is showing the prospective new vet around the practice. James is shown the docking and firing irons (all now obsolete bits of kit) and the emasculators, bloodless castrators and silvery embryotome (all still used in farm practice). Finally, Farnon comes to the fleam, declaring, in all seriousness, "You still can't beat it for laminitis."

My fleam is now on display at *The World of James Herriot*, in Kirkgate, Thirsk, in the museum which was once Herriot's old practice.

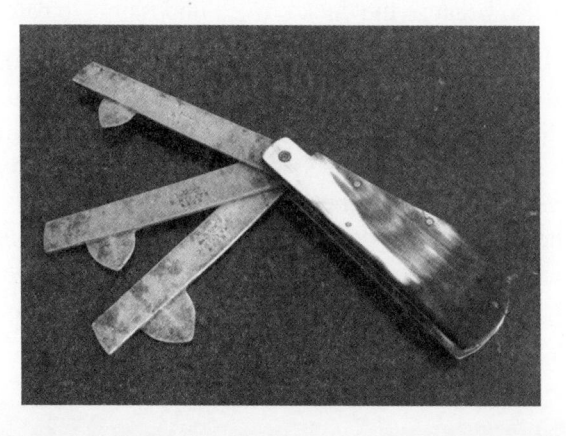

Duck Hunt

Social media can be a great thing, but at times it is exactly the opposite – antisocial media. However, last Saturday it came into its own, as it alerted the animal-loving public (and any off-duty vets in the Thirsk area) to the plight of a duck. A female mallard had been spotted on the banks of Cod Beck near the middle of town, struggling with a fishing line around its leg. I'd just got home and spotted the message on my phone, so called Archie, my youngest son, and we set off, armed with scissors, other cutting implements and some bread for tempting.

"Don't we need a net?" asked Archie, helpfully.

Maybe we did, but I didn't have one. And anyway, I'd done this sort of thing before. In theory, at least, I knew what to do – identify the patient, catch the duck, remove the fishing line. It would surely be easy to spot a lame duck, so to speak. It would surely also be easy to catch a duck who could only hobble. We'd grab it, before it could jump into the river or take to the air. If the duck left terra firma, we had definitely lost our advantage.

The first time I tried to catch a duck was in exactly the same place. A member of the public had called the surgery because he had seen something dangling from the back of the duck. It turned out to be the genitalia, inflamed and swollen, but not in need of any veterinary treatment. Being submerged in cold water was the best cure. This was lucky because there was plenty of cold water to hand and also because the duck proved impossible to catch.

The next time my waterfowl-catching skills were called into action was to aid a swan. This bird, like today's patient, also had a problem with her leg. Remarkably, the swan and her mate had called at the nearest house to their lake and knocked on the door! The birds were clearly asking for help as the female was suffering with a fishing hook in her leg. On that dark, winter's evening almost three years ago, the capture had been hugely successful. Our heroic veterinary

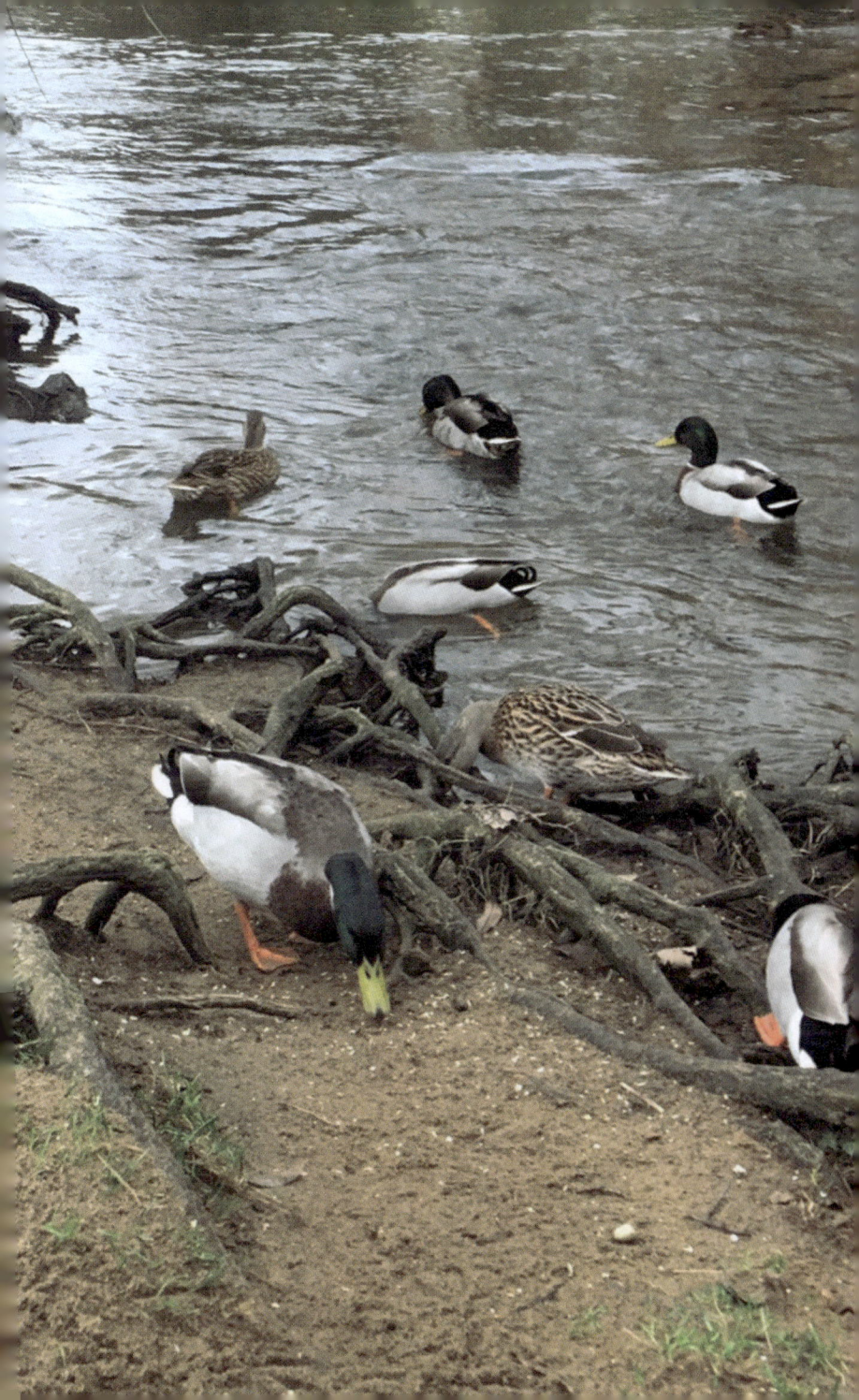

nurse, Sarah, had leapt into the inky lake and grabbed the swan. The fishhook was easily removed, back at the practice safely under general anaesthetic. We kept the swan in the kennels overnight and returned the bird to the lake and to its mate first thing the following morning. The early morning mist floated above the surface of the lake, just like something from the tales of King Arthur. There was no sign of the mate and we worried he might have flown away, traumatised by the nocturnal kidnap of his mate.

But he hadn't. Within just a few moments, he appeared out of the mist and the two swans entwined their necks in a romantic embrace, before floating off together.

But there was no such happy outcome on the banks of Cod Beck this afternoon. The affected duck was nowhere to be seen.

"Some ducks went that way," a helpful dog-walker commented, pointing upstream. We headed in that direction, on another wild duck chase. We found one, sitting near the water's edge, with its feet underwater. It was not moving much and it looked gloomy. Archie made an attempt to grab it. Bad luck again and the duck swam away.

"If one of the legs is tied up, then it will surely swim in circles?" Archie suggested. This one went in a straight line and so did all the others. Gloomily, after almost an hour of searching, we gave up, and ate what was left of the bread. The duck would have to take her chance!

Back to Work

I had spinal surgery a few weeks ago. Before my op, I was worried. Was I doing the right thing? Would the screws go in the right place . . . and what if they didn't? How would I cope with being "out of action" for six whole weeks?

The problem in my back had been developing over some time, but the clinical signs had suddenly become dramatically worse (clinical *signs* are what vets look for to make a diagnosis, as opposed to *symptoms* which are a human patient's description of their problem. Dogs, cats and horses, of course, can't describe their symptoms, so we have to look for the clinical signs. It's a phrase I find hard to abandon). It was clear that something serious needed to be done so, despite my anxieties, seven weeks ago, after my pre-op assessment, I found myself in the prep area, waiting to go into theatre. I could see the surgeon, gloved up and laying out his surgical equipment. It felt all wrong – usually I was holding the scalpel.

At that time, the theatre clock said quarter to nine. The next thing I knew, it was one o'clock and I was wiggling my toes to make sure they still worked. They did and, as I was to discover increasingly over the next few weeks, the operation had been a success. That night, dosed up on morphine, I chatted, giggled and laughed like a loony. The next day I went home. The day after that I walked, slowly and tentatively into Thirsk. It took me twelve and a half minutes. A week later it took me under seven.

I could walk but I couldn't do much else. Moving the coal scuttle was a job too far. I learnt some French (despite the general mood of negativity towards Europe, I love France). I did a bit of writing. I slept on the sofa. I could feel myself recovering. Three weeks later, I went back for a check-up. The surgeon was as delighted as I was with my progress.

But work beckoned. I'd had plenty of messages:

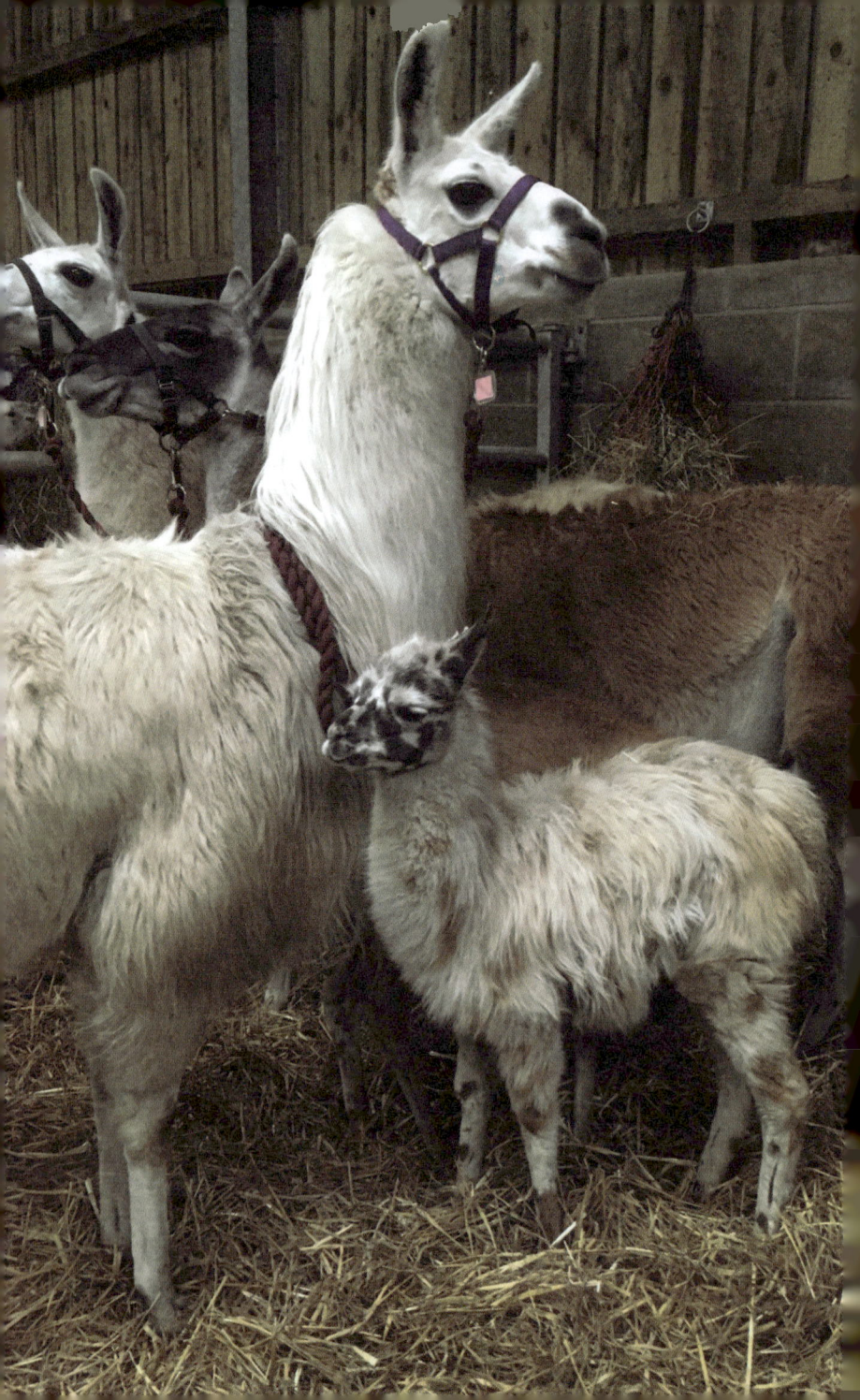

"How are you getting on?"

"When are you back?"

"I'm lambing in January and I'm sure I'll need some help."

"When can you come and see my alpaca?"

"The puppy you delivered by caesarean a couple of months ago needs a first vaccine. When can I come in?"

The messages whetted my appetite to return to work. I missed my patients and their owners, the challenges and rewards of veterinary medicine. But, hard as it was to admit, I was actually quite enjoying some spare time. I'd visited various charities to whom I had promised some time but never managed to find any – Vision 25 in Stockton, a worthy charity supporting adults with disabilities was just one (thank you to Matthew for introducing me to this wonderful place). I was less stressed and my blood pressure was palpably lower. I needed to be back at work, though, as soon as I was able: being a vet.

I know what I'll be doing on my first day back. One job is a llama with an abscess in need of attention. I will pack all my equipment back into the car and head off up to the hills. I can't wait to be back in action. As I write this piece and run my fingers over the precise scars on my lower back, I think about the often-made comparison between vets and medics, ("It's harder to be a vet than a doctor," I hear people say). I am very clear where the true skill lies. It is with the surgeons who can place four life-changing screws with perfect precision into the spine of a human and not with the veterinarian lancing an abscess on the jaw of a llama.

Eating Onions

Anaemia – a deficiency in the body of red blood cells – is a serious condition in both humans and animals. When presented with a case of anaemia, it is essential to work out the cause, even though, at times, this can be complicated. Essentially, it is either due to a reduced rate of production or an increased rate of destruction of red blood cells or their loss from the body through internal or external haemorrhage. Discovering which of these processes is going on is the first step in solving the riddle of anaemia.

Of all the causes of anaemia in dogs and cats, the one that has always stuck in my mind is "Heinz-body anaemia". The red cells are destroyed prematurely because of exposure to a particular type of toxin. You would think, given the name, that the toxin would be something to do with baked beans. It's not though (baked beans are not, to my knowledge, toxic to dogs, although grapes and raisins didn't used to be either, until a few years ago. Now, if the Internet is to be believed, they are amongst some of the most deadly little foodstuffs around).

Heinz bodies are found in the red cells of dogs that have been eating onions. Onions are toxic to dogs, and the oxidative damage they cause to the red cells results in the formation of Heinz bodies and subsequently anaemia as those red cells are destroyed. In some cases, if not diagnosed promptly, it can be fatal. So, when we saw a little dog called Lenny this week, his gums as white as a cricketer's trousers, and with a history of possibly having eaten some onions, Heinz body anaemia was high on the list of possible causes. His owners had been on the Internet and were sure this was the case. However, we could not jump straight to that conclusion and set about some tests. X-rays, abdominal scanning and blood tests quite quickly confirmed that the onions were, in fact, red herrings. Lenny had no Heinz bodies in his cells. He had a bleeding growth on his spleen and before long was in theatre having the offending mass removed.

James, the three-month-old Pug, was the next patient this week to present with suspicious signs. The youngster was walking backwards, which is a very unusual thing for an animal to do. It can indicate severe central brain disease, in the same way as walking around in circles or holding the head in a peculiar position (which he was also doing). Could James have eaten something poisonous or were the signs due to some sort of abnormal development of the young brain? An X-ray showed something in the stomach. James's owner thought he could have eaten a party popper. James, though sad and walking backwards, was not being sick – the usual sign associated with things stuck inside the stomach – so was this another red herring?

He, too, was wheeled into theatre and it would again be a scalpel and not an antidote that came to the rescue. But there was another twist to James's story. The foreign body in his stomach turned out to be not a party popper, but a huge length of un-chewed dog chew, swallowed whole – a painful obstruction as well as a contradiction in terms. The working hypothesis was that the chew (which he had stolen from his mum), and that was jammed across his stomach, was causing so much pain for the poor puppy that he couldn't walk properly or stretch his head down to eat from his bowl. It was an odd theory, but one which, thankfully, turned out to be correct. The following day, James was bombing about the surgery – forwards. For the second time in a week a possible toxicity had proved to be most definitely non-toxic.

Poor James.

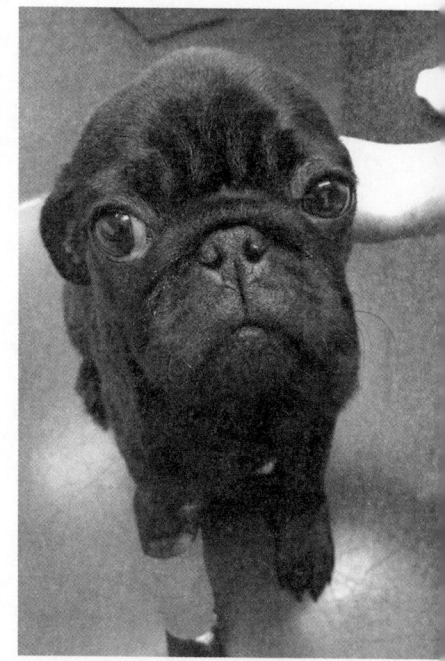

Boris and Luna

We've recently had an addition to our family, in the form of a rescued rabbit. He'd been lost and then found in someone's garden. The finders had scooped him up and taken the lop- eared and slightly droopy rabbit into the surgery to see Anne.

The first job, when faced with a found animal, is to scan it for the presence of a microchip. These grain-of-rice-size devices, despite apparently having the capacity to store a multitude of information, actually just hold a thirteen-digit code, which can be checked against the database via a phone call. The database provides the details of the animal's owner, hopefully allowing them to be reunited. It is most frequently used for cats who've wandered off on an adventure and lost their way or a dog who has strayed from the usual environs of his walk. I had never come across a rabbit who had escaped, got lost and then turned up in another person's garden, but this is what had happened.

"I think I should bring him home – just until we can trace his real owner," said Anne that evening over dinner. "It seems a shame to leave him alone in a kennel all weekend. We have a spare rabbit run and he'd love to spend the weekend out on grass, I'm sure."

It was hard to argue, although I suspected this might be the thin end of a wedge which would result in the lop finding his "forever home" chez Norton. Life was busy. Did we really need another pet?

He arrived that Friday evening and we put him in our spare pen, in sight of our perky little white rabbit, Luna. The new arrival sat, looking around him, clearly confused. The permanent droop of his ears gave him a rather gormless appearance. The kids decided to call him Boris.

As the days went by it became clear that no one was going to come forward to claim Boris. We realised Luna needed a new companion – her previous little friends had gradually flaked out through old age (animals are ephemeral even when owned by two vets). Rabbits are sociable creatures and should not be kept alone. If we could calm him down, reduce his belligerent tendencies, then Boris would make a great companion for the recently bereaved Luna.

Under close supervision, we put the two rabbits together to gauge their reactions. Luna was curious, but Boris made his intentions immediately clear by stomping his feet and then trying to mate with Luna's head. We separated them until we came up with a new plan.

That plan was to castrate him. I looked at Anne – it was surely her turn. I'd castrated our first Border terrier and it was me who spayed Emmy, our Jack Russell. She accepted the challenge immediately (after all, it was Anne who had turned up with the rabbit!) and the following week he was separated from his testicles. We counted down the days required to let his hormones subside before we put them together again. The first day of meeting post-castration was a bit like watching an episode of *Love Island*. We stepped back, watching like voyeurs. They sniffed, hopped and even kissed. But there was no aggression, no stomping of hind feet and certainly no sexual shenanigans. The castration had done the trick and we cautiously continued these bonding sessions over the next few weeks, increasing their length and frequency.

Now, the two rabbits are the very best of friends and utter soulmates. I watch them every day as they sit next to each other, snuggling up and sharing some kale or celery. They spend every minute of every day together, sleeping and cleaning and eating. Boris has certainly landed on his feet and Luna has found her best friend forever.

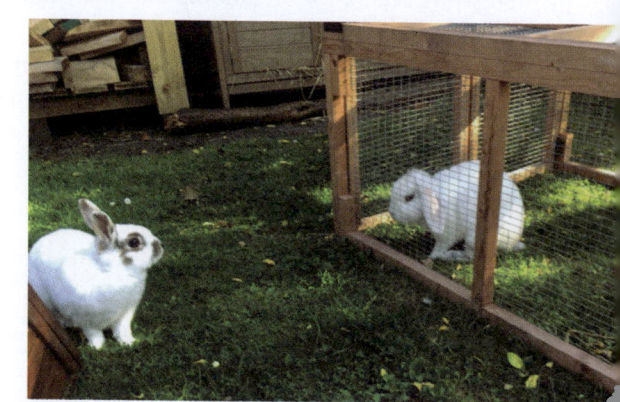

Luna and Boris eye each other up!

Two Crocks

Chris was only slightly apologetic when he called me last week to ask for a bunch of heifers to be dehorned. It was a visit that had been postponed for several months, and now the heifers were large and the job would be strenuous. It would have been much easier to do when the calves were little, but circumstances had conspired against us. We couldn't do it back in the summer, as during warm weather flies take advantage of every minor wound and can wreak havoc. Later in the year, both farmer and vet were out of action, one with a bad back and the other a poorly toe.

We compared X-ray images on our phones before we got down to work with the cattle. Chris's screw was longer than mine, but I had four. Mine seemed to be doing the trick – I proudly explained that I had just had a day's epic mountain biking with my son (although the twinges told me this was probably one adventure too far just a couple of months post op). The long slim screw in Chris's toe wasn't proving quite so effective and he was awaiting another appointment with the surgeon.

As such, the two crocks set about what should have been the relatively simple job of removing twelve medium-sized horns from six medium-sized animals. The moving of the gates was a bit like an episode of the Chuckle Brothers. We struggled and hobbled to hoist them into place, but this was the easy bit, because next we had to persuade the heifers into the small pen that we had just made. This involved a lot of shooing and waving. As farm work goes, it was not particularly dangerous: the cattle were not belligerent nor trying to cause any trouble. But our reactions needed to be quick, because if they tried to run past us we would be at risk of being knocked over and trampled. A farmer with a painful toe, limping even on the flat ground of his farmyard, and a vet with a newly screwed-together lumbar spine, did not make a dream team.

Chris tripped over a pile of bedding and landed flat on his face. He got up cursing and laughing. I cursed that I didn't have a camera following me around today! We worked steadily, within our limits and eventually the job was completed, relatively uneventfully. Dehorning cattle is not my favourite job, but it had all gone smoothly. I recalled to Chris one of the hardest sessions I'd had, many years ago at a farm just outside Ampleforth. I was there to TB-test a small herd of about thirty cows. This would have been half a morning's job on its own, but the farmer wanted to take advantage of having a vet on his farm and asked me to dehorn almost the entire herd, every member of which was replete with horns of wild-west proportions. Each horn was about as wide at its base as a gin and tonic glass. By cow number twenty-five, and hence horn number fifty, I was flagging and (for the first and only time in my veterinary life) asked the farmer's son, who was about eighteen and helping, if he could do a couple, just until I regained some strength.

He did one horn, huffing and puffing and sweating like a tap, before throwing in his towel. "It's too hard for me!" he gasped, and left me to finish the job. I was a tired man by the end of the day and missed my appointment at the gym that evening. Thinking back, there's no real wonder my back is jiggered!

The bull looks on as I remove horns.

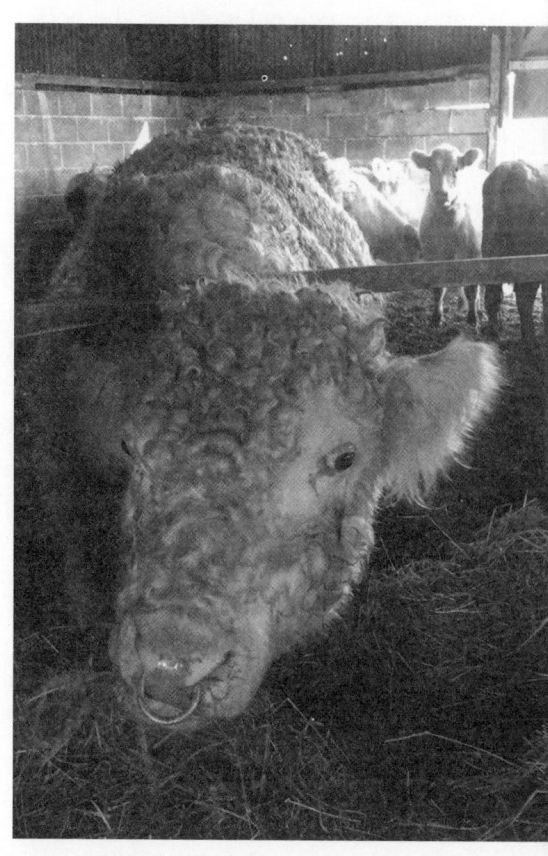

Alpacas on the Telly

Last week was busier and more unusual than most. The first part of my week was filled with the standard cats, dogs and even the odd ferret needing attention. There were farm visits to rush to and urgent operations. But, on Thursday, my next book was published – *A Yorkshire Vet: The Next Chapter*. I really should apologise for writing so many books, but I really like it. The process of drawing stories from the back of my mind and putting them to paper (via a laptop) is both rewarding and cathartic and I seem to have developed something of an obsessive and compulsive passion for writing. This is my fifth book in as many years. My publishers – the mighty Hodder and Stoughton, whose headquarters is possibly bigger and more impressive than any building I have ever been inside – had arranged some publicity for the book. This necessitated another trip to London: I had an appointment with Phillip and Holly and they had requested alpacas! It would be a far cry from my usual veterinary antics in Yorkshire.

The alpacas took some arranging. Luckily, I have a few good friends in the camelid world with useful connections. Before long and after only about ten emails, I managed to find a well-behaved and local pair to go, with their owners, to Television Centre, Wood Lane, London. I recognised the address, because it was the same one that I used to write to when I entered a *Blue Peter* competition, or to where I would send collected stamps for an appeal to save something or help someone. But that was when I was ten.

So, on Thursday morning, some alpacas and I arrived at the "talent" entrance of this famous place. Spitfire was friendly and composed, but somewhat aloof. Pete and I, however, hit it off like a pair of kindred spirits. As the friendly alpaca and I chatted in advance of our debut on *This Morning*, I suspected there might be fireworks on set before too long. The alpacas went first, for an introduction to the famous TV presenters and to benefit from a rehearsal. I didn't get to rehearse and I'm not sure why. Did they think I was a TV pro?

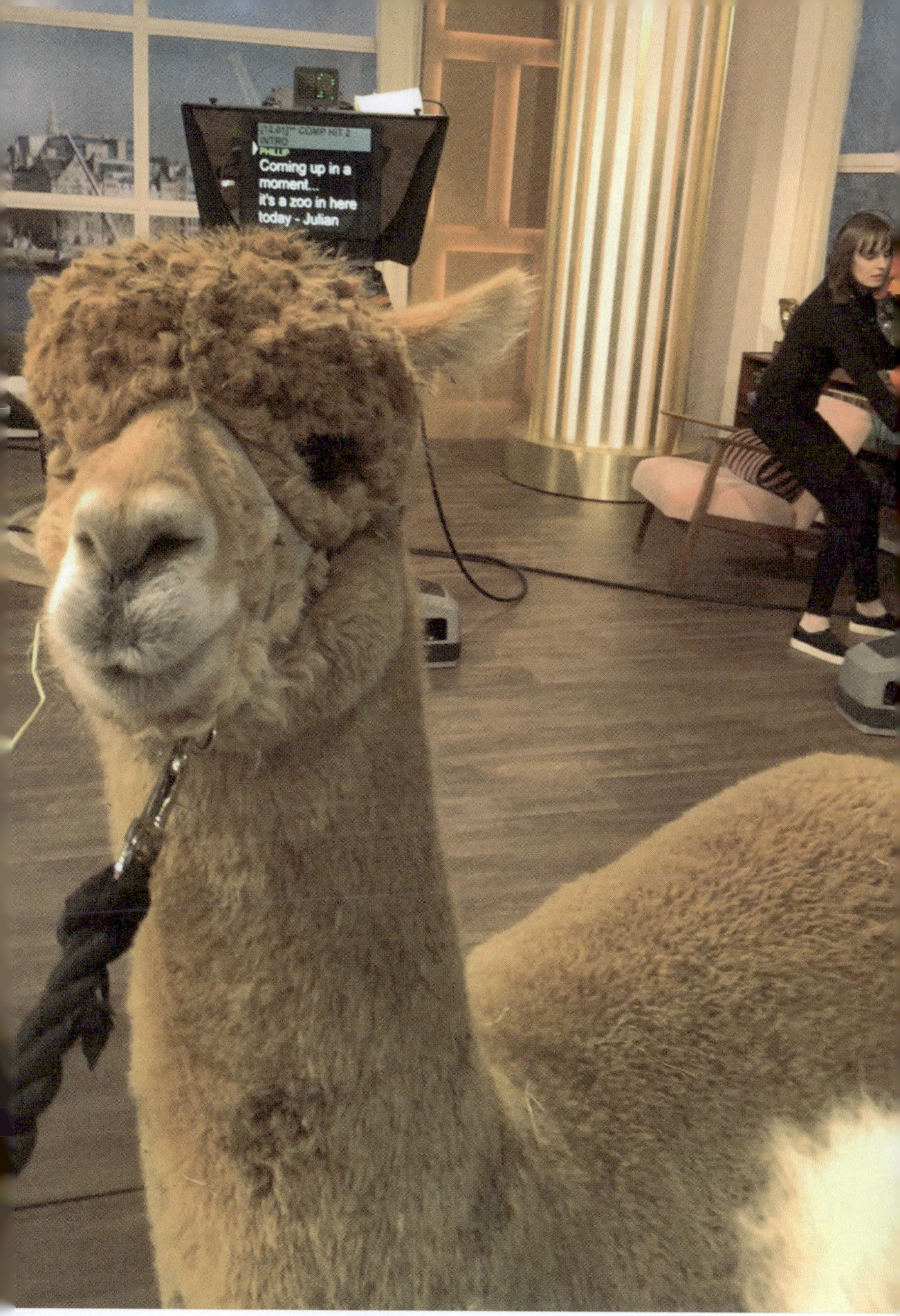
INTRO
Coming up in a moment...
it's a zoo in here today - Julian

But my lack of rehearsal did not matter, because it was not me that took centre stage. My new bestie Pete the alpaca took that honour. Within minutes of the animals meeting Holly and Phillip, tension developed. Holly is notoriously nervous around animals (they had a pig on the previous day and he had also caused havoc) and she stayed at a safe distance. Phillip, for his part, was not nervous but, despite his role as Dr Dolittle in the West End production, was evidently reasonably inept around animals. He pulled on their lead ropes as Holly observed from afar. Pete sensed the unease and spat directly into the multi-award-winning presenter's face, causing much amusement to the production team. Holly collapsed on the floor in helpless giggles.

Luckily composure was soon regained by all. Phillip wiped the spit off his face and Pete calmed down. Minutes later, I was called into action, holding onto the alpacas and acting as referee. We talked, live on national telly, as naturally as if we were standing waiting for a bus or having a drink in the pub. Me, a Yorkshire vet, holding and reassuring two alpacas, along with possibly the two most famous telly presenters of recent times. I had to pinch myself because it was hard to believe. But the glamorous world of green rooms and celebs would be short-lived. On Friday, I had farmers to see and dogs to fix and life would be normal again.

Chateauneuf du Hamster

It had been another long day, with operations in the morning and visits to see horses and llamas in the afternoon. There were lots of llamas, too. One had a sore leg; he'd been running in the mud and strained a ligament in his stifle (an injury usually seen in overactive spaniels and football players). Another was suffering from a lumpy face, which I hoped was an abscess and nothing more sinister, and third was losing condition despite eating like a horse, necessitating blood and faecal samples. And, as usual, there was a check-up on the enigmatic llama with the heart murmur, which I always had a listen to, just to make sure things hadn't changed or deteriorated too much. Then there was a half-hour drive back to Boroughbridge, to tackle evening surgery. After that, it was home time, although it was hard to call it "home time" because I was on call. If an emergency reared its head I might not be at home for very long. Depending when that emergency appeared, I might not even get home!

Evening surgery was uneventful and the idea of a nice meal and some time with the family or sitting on the sofa watching TV was gradually filling my thoughts. But it was not to be. At least not just yet, because there was one final patient, added to the end of my list. It was a hamster.

I really like hamsters, mainly because of their endless energy and constant enthusiasm, which is hard not to admire. Not all vets, however, are keen on these little mammals, because they have a bad habit of sinking their sharp and long incisors into the fingers of those who prod them, and not letting go. Within the profession, there are salutary tales of vets who, in an attempt to remove a hamster dangling angrily from a pinky, have shaken their hand so vigorously that the poor creature has been flung across the consulting room. It has never happened to me, but I retain a healthy respect for these feisty little mammals.

The hamster on this evening's list was, as usual, called Hammy. He

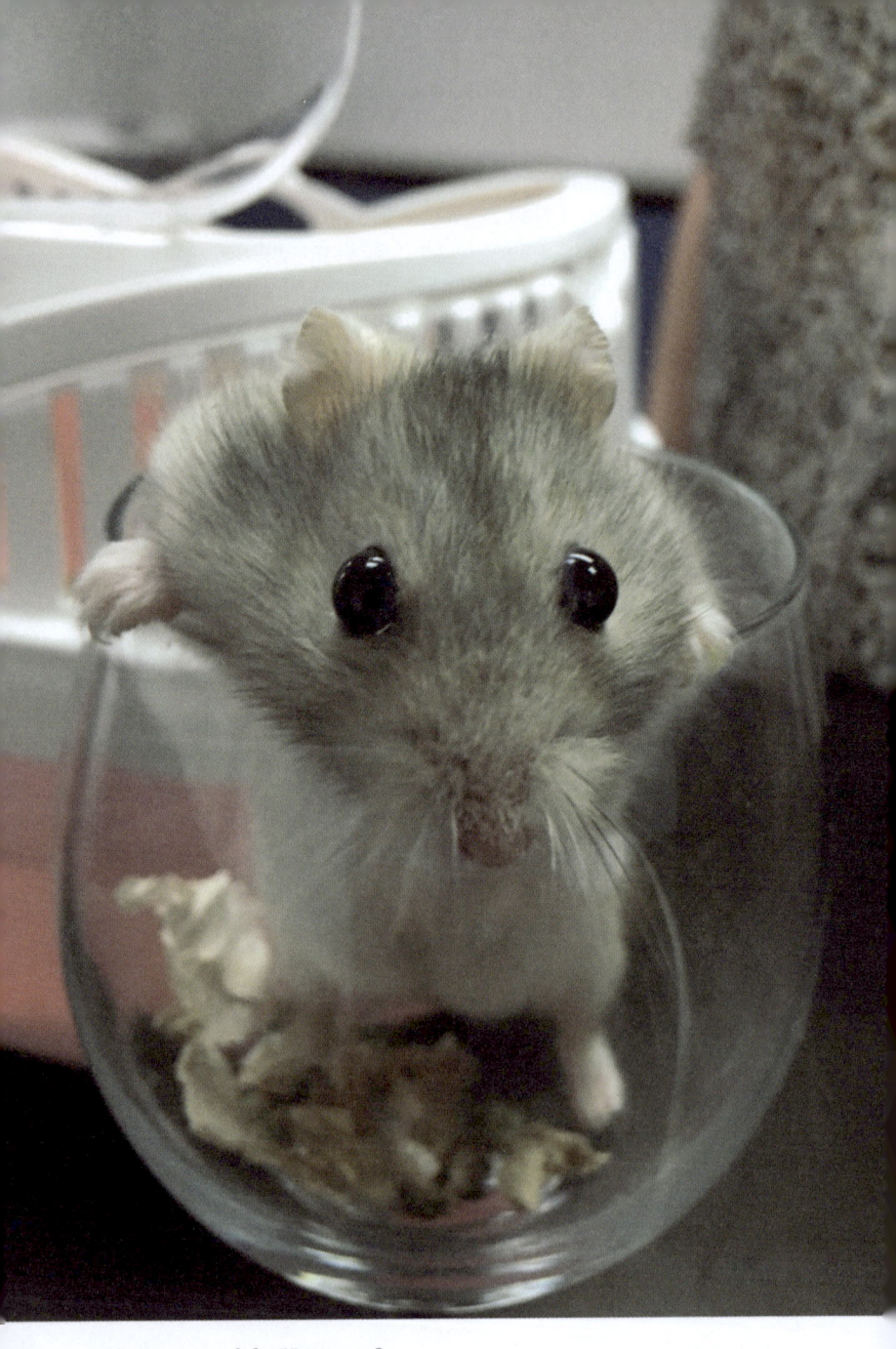

Chateauneuf du Hamster?

had a sore tummy – or, at least, some sort of swelling or bulging lump on his underside. As I peered into the shoebox that was acting as a pet carrier and watched him scuttle around the sawdust, I wondered how I was going to manage an effective examination. Then I had a brilliant idea. I'm not sure if it was because my mind swings towards the idea of wine once the clock has chimed six on a Friday evening, but I found myself rummaging in a cupboard in the kitchen at the practice for a wine glass. The cupboard is mostly full of coffee mugs and biscuits, but I'd spotted a couple of glasses, presumably either for special occasions at the practice or for desperate vets. Anyhow, I returned from the cupboard to the consulting room, triumphantly clutching the glass. I scooped Hammy up in it and raised him, not so much as a toast, but more so I could safely inspect his undercarriage. It worked a treat. The glass could have almost been designed for the purpose. Hammy had a patch of dermatitis on his tummy and nothing worse. I prescribed some ointment and took my customary photograph (I take photos of anything vaguely interesting/amusing/cute/gooey these days), before returning the little dude to his shoebox. I was soon out of the door and heading for the comfort and relaxation of my sofa, and it would not be long before I had another wine glass well and truly in my hand. This time though, it would be full of Cote du Rhone and not Chateauneuf-du-Hamster.

Coronavirus. Or Actual Facts

So here's a thing. Cats get coronavirus. Of course, it is not the same as human coronavirus and it causes a completely different disease to the one humans can get, the one which is currently causing global chaos. The disease feline coronavirus can cause is called *Feline Infectious Peritonitis*. If you have a cat, do not panic. There is no need to enforce quarantine or lock it in the shed. Having recently returned from the French Alps (where, I think, one case was identified three weeks ago), my wife has been banned from her Pilates class – metaphorically also locked in the shed. Is this a sound precaution or an annoying inconvenience and upon what information was it based, given that she did the NHS online survey and came out all clear?

As I write, I am listening to a radio programme and the host of the phone-in is asking for doctors and healthcare officials to call. It seems there is a dearth of proper information there, too. Thankfully an emergency doctor has called in. He has some facts, some actual facts. The presenter of the programme is now stuck. She doesn't know what to do when faced with someone with proper data. It turns out coronavirus is worse than standard flu. Its virulence factor (the number of new cases which are generated per clinical case, i.e. a measure of how infectious the disease is) is 2.2. This is about twice that of influenza. That means that the new coronavirus is about twice as infectious as standard 'flu.

From the doctor on the radio, more facts quickly follow. The mortality rate (the percentage of clinical cases which die) is approximately one per cent. The death rate from 'flu is 0.1 per cent, so this coronavirus is, so far, about ten times as deadly as flu. These figures sound fairly bad, but in total, global terms, the actual health impact of the apparently novel virus has, so far, been low. However, there is one absolute certainty: that the virus *will* spread worldwide before too long. Airborne viruses are brilliant at spreading. A disease like HIV back in the 1980s, was spread by certain very specific routes. If you avoid those activities, you stood little chance of contracting that particular infection. But with an upper respiratory disease it is surely close to impossible to halt its spread.

But we need not to panic, nor should we. (I studied virology as an extra degree during my veterinary course at Cambridge, so I am qualified to talk about this). Although there is no proper cure for viral infections, their Achilles heel is that a virus particle relies entirely on a relationship with a cell to multiply and survive. A virus that kills its host, whether it's a cat or a human, has no hope of surviving. In short, it's not a very good virus if it kills its host. Most viruses attenuate their pathogenicity over time, which is why virus outbreaks start dramatically and then peter out. Think of the major virus outbreaks over recent history. None of them trivial, but the inexorable expansion of the world's population has not yet been dented. And, like small children returning from the toilet, or from playing in the mud, fully grown adults, who are hopefully already aware of basic hygiene, are told to wash our hands and save the world.

Back in the veterinary clinic, life continues in a non-panicky way and we only wear facemasks when cleaning dirty dogs' teeth or mixing up chemotherapy drugs (both happened on Friday last week. I was tempted to post on Instagram, but refrained for fear of inducing more panic). I'm just really, really hoping I don't have to diagnosis a cat with peritonitis and tell its owner their cat has coronavirus. But, of course, if I did, I'd furnish them with all the actual facts.

Hedgehog Three Legs

The ops list last Friday was full of cats to spay, Labradors with lumps to remove and investigations into vomiting dogs and wheezing cats. There was also a rabbit with a weepy eye to deal with. But the procedure everyone in the practice wanted to watch was the case of Mrs Tiggywinkle, who was a pet albino hedgehog. Like her eponymous namesake, the hedgehog had become a superstar since her arrival in the waiting room a week or so before. Even though the injury to her left front leg was serious, and being able to fix it was by no means guaranteed, nurses and vets alike were stealing selfies with this super cute creature.

I knew the challenge would be considerable, but I was soon to discover that there was an added pressure. It turned out that Mrs Tiggywinkle's owner was a toddler of nearly three years old, who had just got the hang of conversation and was full of empathy for his favourite little spiky pet. I had met him earlier in the morning.

"She's got a poorly leg," said Zac carefully, as he plonked the cardboard box at his head height, onto the table in front of him. He picked his nose and tried to climb up onto the table, as only toddlers can. The injured leg was, as Zac had described, very poorly. In fact, the foot was becoming necrotic. There was only one option and that was to amputate said poorly leg. I was anxious about the anaesthetic and how the surgery would go, but I dared not contemplate the reaction of Zac, or the deflation of our staff, if Mrs T did not make it through.

I've amputated countless bits of animals in my career and it's never a nice thing to do. It is always a last resort. Vets try to save things – lives and limbs – and so amputating a leg, or a tail, or a toe is a last resort and usually only employed when a cat has sustained an irreparably smashed limb under a fast-moving car or a dog has a cancerous bone. In theory, amputating a hedgehog's leg would be similar process, but a new procedure on a novel patient always raises the pulse.

I had considered how Mrs T would cope with just three legs. Generally, four-legged creatures manage just fine with a twenty-five percent reduction in the number of weight-bearing limbs. I'd seen many three-legged hedgehogs rescued from the wild, after accidents with garden netting or pieces of entwined string. They always seemed perfectly capable. If the worst came to the worst, I reasoned, Mrs T could simply become ball-shaped and roll along.

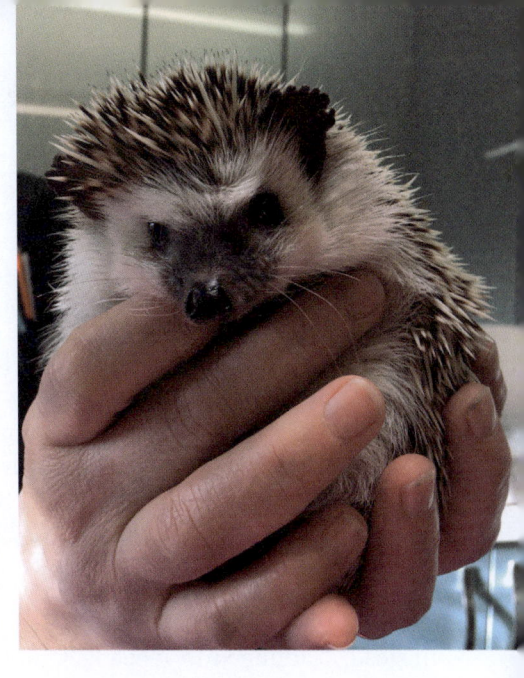

But that turned out not to be necessary. The anaesthetic – tense for just a while (Fiona, the nurse kept things stable and calm) – was smooth and the surgery uneventful. Before long, Mrs Tiggywinkle was recovered and quickly assumed a spherical pose. At the end of the busy day, her owners reappeared to collect her. Mrs Tiggywinkle was delighted that her son's favourite albino hedgehog had made it through the tricky procedure, but not as delighted as young Zac. Unaware of exactly the magnitude of what had just happened, he was, nevertheless, delighted to be reunited with his pet and celebrated by delving into a plastic bag and dropping a toddler-sized handful of cat food and mealworms in front of Mrs T. She unrolled and immediately tucked into the tasty morsels.

I was happy with a good job done, not just because I hoped I'd saved Mrs T's spiky skin, but because it had made a little boy very happy. Before he left, he thanked me and promptly thrust out his cat-foody hand for me to shake. It had been a good day.

Reel Around the Fountain

My first appointment of the afternoon sounded clandestine.

At half past two Jack, the "Somethingapoo", needed his regular and life preserving injection. Jack had a serious illness that necessitated monthly injections. He also had a needle phobia.

The solution, according to the dog behaviourist, was to meet at a venue remote from the veterinary surgery, thus avoiding the negative association between the surgery and the injection. A plan had been hatched between Jack's owner and one of the nurses, to meet in a car park somewhere between Boroughbridge and Scotton. In theory, at least, this was a sound plan. In practice, I had no intention of meeting a lady and her fluffy dog in a random car park. If spotted, people might talk.

Instead, I arranged to meet Jack and his owner in the middle of Boroughbridge, next to the fountain. It isn't actually a fountain because no water comes out of it. It looks more like a small and therefore useless bandstand. Nevertheless, it made a convenient rendezvous point. I spotted Jack, waiting beside a bench with his owner, who was armed with a large block of cheese – apparently the weapon of choice advised by canine behavioural therapists. The idea was that the tasty cheese would distract the dog from his fear of needles. Small morsels of sausage also, apparently, work. I was armed with a small syringe filled with Jack's powerful medicine.

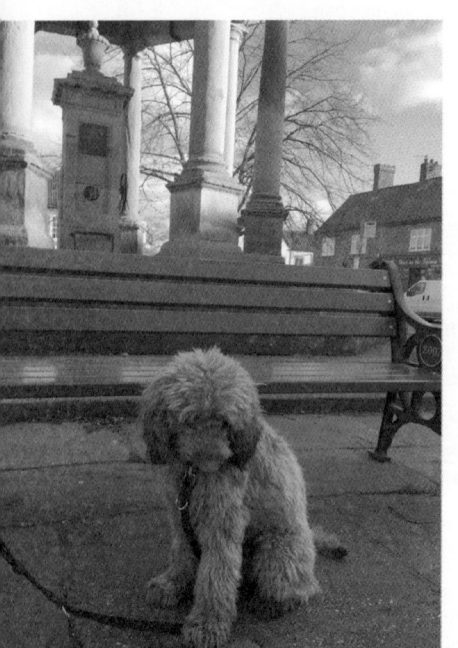

We met, chatted, ruffled ears and ate crumbs of Cheddar on the bench, before getting down to business.

In the "olden days" (in my third decade of practice, I think I am just about entitled to use this phrase) there was a superb tablet for treating Jack's illness. It came in stumpy brown glass bottles, each with an unassuming khaki and white label. Each bottle held, inexplicably, just thirty little, life-saving tablets. Given that most dogs would need between five and ten tablets per day, each bottle lasted less than a week, which was not very environmentally friendly. The recycling bin filled very quickly. Despite its diminutive packaging and its benign name (it was full of soft letters like "f"s), this drug kept many dogs with this unusual condition alive and healthy. Sadly, it was discontinued and a new drug was produced with a sexy name, full of "z"s. Modern, sexy drugs nearly all have names including lots of "z"s, "x"s and "v"s. This particular one comes only as an injection, which is even more sexy if you're a pharmaceutical company, but not if you are a needle-phobic dog like Jack. What the behaviourist had failed to take into account was that a needle is a needle, whether it is in the surgery, in a car park or by the fountain. Even though Jack was calm and free from the stress of the vet clinic, he quickly realised what I was up to and spun around intent on avoiding my syringe. I must have administered hundreds of thousands of injections to animals over my career and, I have to say, I'm pretty good at it. The medicine was injected safely and effectively, but poor Jack was rolling on the ground in apparent distress for some minutes afterwards. Even cheese did not bring an early end to his anguish. The plan had clearly not worked at all and I did not fancy any more al fresco meetings like this, cheese or no cheese.

"You know, there might be another way." I suddenly had a flash of inspiration. "There is an old tablet that we used to use for treating this condition. If you can find any on-line you should get as much as you can. Then he wouldn't need any more injections." I hoped there were some out there somewhere. Sometimes the old treatments are the best.

Rescued from a Spanish Ravine

Meg the dog was in for what was, on the face of it, a simple consultation. She was a new patient to the practice and needed her vaccinations, including those required to allow her to travel to and from continental Europe for a forthcoming family holiday. In amongst the chaos of Brexit, vets were given regular, but often quickly obsolete, updates by DEFRA regarding how the regulations for the travel arrangements for cats, dogs and – amusingly – ferrets might change. I have completed hundreds of pet passports over the years but, disappointingly, I have never, ever come across a travelling ferret. I wish I had. It would make a great story – maybe one day I will write a book entitled *Travelling Europe with a Ferret*, based on the adventures of said creature and me, a bit like Tony Hawks' book about hitching around Ireland with a fridge.

But this is beside the point and not the topic of today's article, which is Meg.

Meg was apparently very healthy, but she looked unusual because her ears had been "clipped". This cosmetic procedure was banned in Britain many years ago so it is not something we see often. Clipping the ears involved cutting off the folding over part of the ear-flap. The result is that the ears look permanently pricked to attention, and the dog looks unusually and persistently alert.

"Meg is from Spain," her owner explained, as I looked puzzled, partly because of her odd, non-UK ears, and partly because her vaccination certificate was in a language I did not understand. Only our once communal ring of golden stars on a dark blue background demonstrated a previous common allegiance.

"My husband found her in Spain. She was stranded at the bottom of a ravine. We think she'd fallen in and couldn't get out."

From the same folder as Meg's Spanish vaccination certificate, her owner produced a photo album containing photographs of Meg at various stages throughout her rescue and recuperation. The

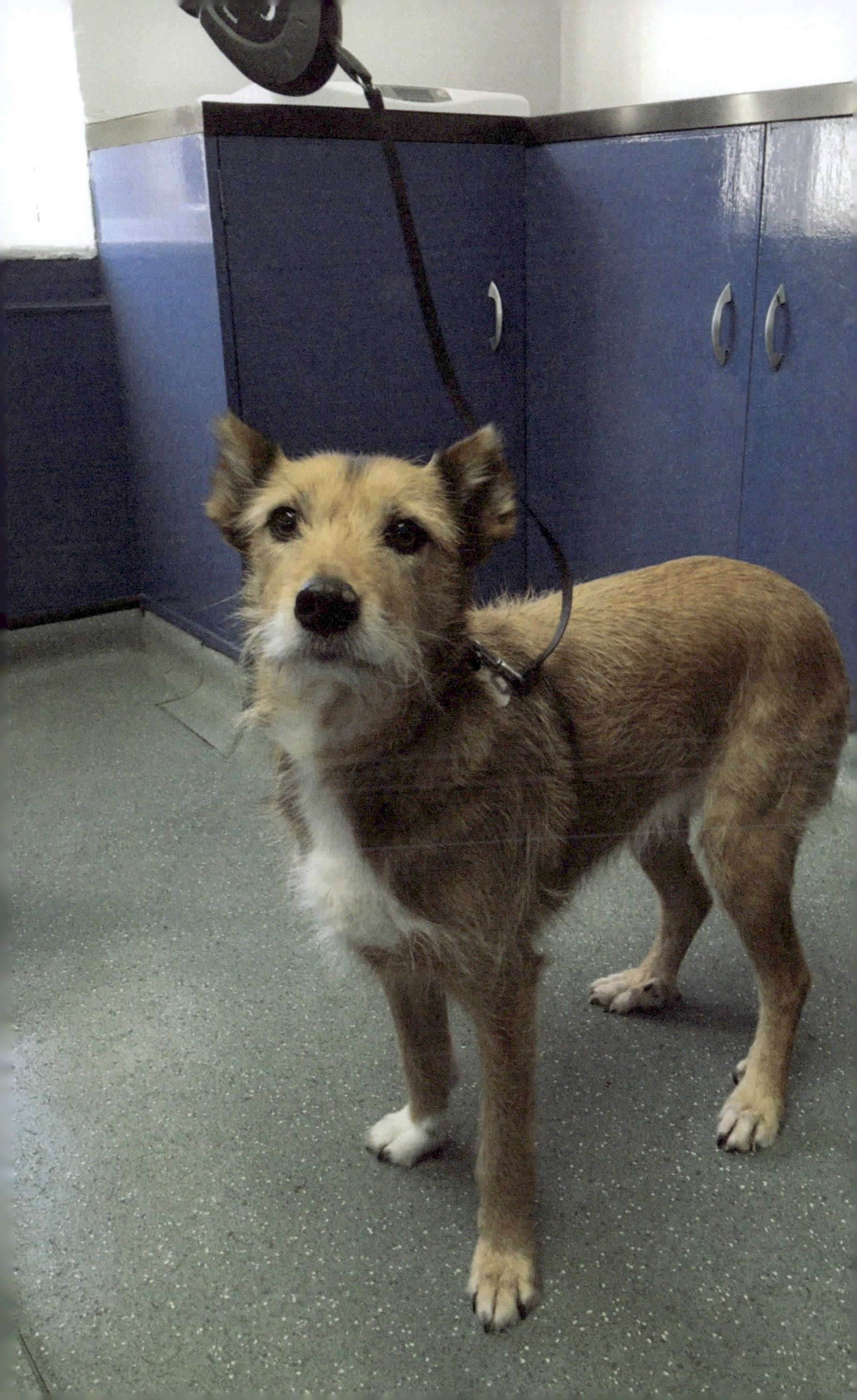

consultation had changed from a clinical examination to an episode of *This Is Your Life* and brought parts of *The Lion King* to mind.

"And he climbed in, not knowing how he would catch her, let alone lift her out. He didn't know if she was rabid or fierce. It turned out she was neither and now she's our pet and has lived with us ever since."

We marvelled at the stoicism of animals and how some really did seem to land on their feet. I could not claim any stories of similar drama, but I do have some friends who recently rescued a street cat from Tbilisi, the capital of the Caucasian country of Georgia. This cat, who is called Mtatsie, is as relaxed and content as any cat could be, having also landed on his feet and moved from the dusty mountainous area between Europe and Asia to his permanent home surrounded by alpine pastures in France, via Portsmouth.

Meg was fit and well, so I administered the appropriate vaccines and made the required additions to her pet passport to confirm her health and suitability to travel. Apparently, she revisited Spain regularly with her owners and was a seasoned traveller. After the Brexit issue, vets have finally received some temporarily accurate information about pet travel in the post-Brexit apocalypse. There has been much speculation about whether this would even remain possible. Happily, for Meg, Mtatsie and hundreds of dogs and cats all over the UK, the big news has been confirmed: nothing will change! At least, not until the end of 2020. Although in the current global crisis who knows, even the ferrets, when any of us will be free to use our passports ever again.

It's You-thanasia

A visit to put a dog to sleep was scheduled as my last job on Saturday morning. It was an elderly Labrador, who had been struggling with mobility for some time. Eventually the medicines had stopped giving her any relief and Ellie's owners were forced to make the final decision. Once morning surgery had finished, I telephoned to confirm the time and to talk through that decision. I also needed to get accurate directions to the house, which I scribbled on a scrap of paper – past the felled tree on the left, right at the corner by the house with vertical panels on its fence, down a lane and then right at the "fancy" sign. Their house was at the end of the lane. The last detail was that it was the white house on the right, but my paper was too small to fit this on. The rest of the information was so specific that I felt sure I'd find the premises without a problem.

I gathered my equipment in a small plastic bag – a swab to clean the leg where the injection would go, two syringes of strong barbiturate and my trusty curved scissors to snip away hair from the front leg so I could see the vein where the injection would be given. Armed with these and the directions, I headed out for my least favourite type of visit. Putting down animals is the worst part of the job for a vet. The only mitigating factor, which makes it bearable, is that it's usually being done for the right reasons: intractable pain or incurable illness. The relief to a sick patient is immediate, although it almost always takes some time for the grieving owner to share that relief. Ellie's owner was certain the time was right to say goodbye but this didn't make the sad job any easier.

I passed the felled tree and the directions were perfect. I turned right at the fancy sign and pulled up on the pebbled drive outside the imposing front door of the house at the end of the long lane and grabbed my stethoscope along with my bag of kit. I knocked on the door and, seeing a lady walking towards me, opened it and went into the large, farmhouse kitchen.

"Oh, hello!" she said, sounding surprised. "Well, I've just been reading your piece in the *Yorkshire Post* about the dog who had a phobia of needles!"

"Oh, yes," I replied, suddenly remembering that people actually do read these columns, a fact that is easy to put to the back of the mind when composing each one at the kitchen table late on an evening.

"I really hope *your* dog isn't needle-phobic today!" I added to try to lift what would surely be a sombre mood.

"Why do you say that?" the lady said, now sounding confused as well as surprised.

"Well, I've come to put down your dog," I explained, lifting my bag of lethal injection.

"Oh, dear. I think you've got the wrong house!" I went cold. "My dogs are out with my husband at the moment, on a walk. They're both very healthy."

I was mortified. Not only had I walked into someone's kitchen uninvited, but I'd also suggested I was about to euthanise a perfectly healthy family pet. Luckily, the house-owner was amused rather than offended and I was pointed in the direction of the *white* house on the *right*, just a hundred yards away, where an elderly Labrador and an anxious owner were waiting patiently. I apologised profusely for being late and explained my story. Despite the tears of sadness, Ellie's owner couldn't help but laugh. "Well," she said, "I think you've got a good story to write about in next week's column!"

Life in a Time of Corona 1

It would be an understatement to say that this has been an interesting week. Following the announcement by the government last week, everyone's life is very different. Advice from our professional bodies has been read and digested and various meetings have been called. A profession which simply cannot work from home has vigorously embraced Skype and FaceTime.

I pondered my recent weekend on call, the one that came just before the apocalyptically named "LOCKDOWN" was announced. As is always the case in spring, it was busy. A dog with a broken leg, sustained when it failed to clear a cattle grid, could not be treated over the phone, or from home. The four sheep to lamb and the alpaca with a prolapse all required hands-on attention and so too did a pyrexic dog with prostatitis, which needed intravenous antibiotics throughout Saturday evening and most of Sunday. So, it is fortunate that vets are still allowed to continue our work, at least to some extent. After lengthy discussion, a plan was hatched. A plan of sorts, but one which attempted to balance the requirement to provide care for patients in need, protect the public and protect ourselves, or at least minimise our risks. Over the subsequent days, it was fascinating to see how these, sometimes conflicting, priorities would play out. The front door was shut and clients had to wait outside; routine procedures were cancelled. But then, what constitutes a routine procedure? The puppy, for instance, who has started his vaccination course and who would be homebound for an unspecified period of time if he didn't receive his second injection – surely it would be better to finish the course? But did it count as routine? Best veterinary practice had to be modified – could we really achieve an adequate diagnosis by a phone call or a photo on an email?

In the case of Babs the bald guinea pig, I was happy to make a sound judgement following both these things. An avoided visit to the clinic is another exercise in social distancing. We are told to minimise human-to-human contact "to stop the spread of this invisible threat." In reality, the bigger risk is *to* our clients rather than *from* them. Like other people working directly with the public, vets are certain to be at an increased risk of exposure. And it's almost impossible to keep our distance. I couldn't ask each farmer I'd seen over the weekend to "stand a broom-length away" otherwise the sheep would have run off, never to be lambed!

Given that COVID-19 is so ubiquitous and infectious (and nobody knows its true prevalence because so little testing has been done) becoming infected seems just a matter of time for all of us. To try to mitigate the problems that this will bring, part of our plan at work has been to split into two teams, working separately and independently of one another. Should one of us succumb, the other team can continue to work in health and harmony, avoiding the need to close down the whole practice. I am in team B, which is smaller but arguably more perfectly formed. I wasn't around at team selection, but I imagine it was a bit like when football teams were chosen at school. Who would be the last to get picked?

I returned to base to find the team selection had been completed. There was just one vet's car in the practice – belonging to my teammate. I presumed the two of us were starting the first shift. But no! On the day of inception of our "team play" policy, ALL of the A team had been dispatched within five minutes of each other. Two were doing a caesarean on a cow and the third was repairing a prolapsed ewe! So much for working from home!

Life in a Time of Corona 2

We are still getting used to our compromised work situation. I had said goodbye to half of the practice – those in team A. We commiserated over a tray bake and coffee and I checked everyone's temperature one last time. My infrared thermometer had been a godsend, as much for peace of mind as for making a diagnosis. The first time I'd seen such a nifty device was when a friend checked the temperature inside her newly built pizza oven. It needed to be at a minimum of three hundred degrees for perfect pizzas and the thermometer could give a reading just by aiming into the glowing embers. It turns out, there is a similar device for taking the temperature of humans. I was in hospital a few months ago for back surgery and, every hour or so, a nurse would appear and point the medical equivalent at my forehead. A green light and a smiley baby face would confirm that my temperature was okay. If it was aimed at the side of a mug of tea, a red light and a frowning baby would appear on the digital display screen. The device was left beside my bed and it captivated my morphine-fuelled attention. I picked it up and tested it on various parts of my body, concluding it worked on gums and lips. I decided to get one of these and see if it worked on animals. If it did, the instant results without the need for rectal intrusion might revolutionise the veterinary world. Sadly, this did not transpire to be the veterinary breakthrough I had hoped for and the results on dogs were hopelessly inaccurate. Until life in a time of coronavirus, it was a redundant piece of equipment but now it is worth its weight in gold. I checked my temperature multiple times every morning and that of anyone else who asked.

Everyone's temperatures were normal and we parted, afebrile but without hugs, pondering what would happen to the workload over the next few weeks and how we'd cope. There had been suggestions of conducting consultations through the window of the consulting room, for example. I'd suggested we could perform kennel cough vaccinations (which require a dose to be administered up the dog's nose) through the letter box of the front door. Nobody found my attempt to lighten the mood very funny. Evaluating what sort of work constitutes an emergency and is therefore acceptable under the COVID-19 clampdown can be complicated. It has, so far, been very interesting to see how each case is judged on its merit and how vets have different views. Obviously, we follow our professional guidelines but, as with most lines, there can be some blurring as conflicting needs are balanced. A kennel cough vaccination, for example, seems a non-essential veterinary job under the circumstances, until you realise that it gives peace of mind to the elderly owner, worried in case she has to go to hospital and her dog might be refused access to kennels.

Clients have been, so far, very accommodating to our requests to distance themselves from us, although I constantly find myself apologising for leaving people standing in the street! One client though, was thoroughly indignant when it was explained that clipping a dog's nails did not count as an emergency. The owner of a rabbit, whose vaccination would need to be put on hold for a few weeks was equally offended.

"But that means I'll have to keep him inside," she protested. "He'll be very cross about that!" I refrained from replying the obvious: that the rabbit could join the rest of the club.

Life in a Time of Corona 3

As the practice busied itself to cope with providing as normal a service as possible, with limited staff and even more limited contact with the public, our two teams went their separate ways. Team A were first on the rota.

I was in Team B, so I stocked up my car, ready for my next stint and gathered some paperwork and reading to do at home. I pondered leaving my magic thermometer, so that everyone could keep a check on their temperatures, but given the degree of scepticism of its reliability from my colleagues, and my recently formed habit of twice-daily measurements, I decided to keep hold of it. As I drove back up the A168, with a good couple of hours of daylight left, I started to plan my daily quota of exercise. I could get out on my bike from home, through Upsall, up Sneck Yate and back via Whitehorse Bank before darkness fell.

But by the time I pulled up the drive, an unusual and unfamiliar inertia had set in. Suddenly, the idea of toiling up one of Yorkshire's steepest roads did not seem appealing. I pointed the magic thermometer at my forehead again and noted the reading was a couple of decimal places higher than it had been earlier in the day. Was it just the thick fleece I was wearing? I peeled off a couple of layers and rechecked half an hour later. It had gone up again, by another 0.2 degrees. For now, I kept quiet and stayed inside. By the middle of the evening the reading had risen to the point where the green light with the smiling picture of a baby's face had changed to a red light and a frowning baby. I didn't feel particularly ill, nor did I fear imminent hospitalisation, but I knew I was not right. I told Anne, who was more worried than me, and I sent a message to a colleague, promising to reassess with more information and a plan by morning.

By morning I was properly hot. The NHS website advice was pretty clear. I needed to stay at home for a week. My family needed to stay inside for two – which meant Anne couldn't go to work either. I called the practice, apologising profusely for upsetting the rota. Everyone seemed happy for me to stay away, especially when I explained the soreness of my throat, the mild headache and developing tracheal cough, which sounded like a terrier with kennel cough. The next thing I knew, it was half past one in the afternoon and I'd missed the morning, fast asleep in bed. This was not a normal thing. I felt sure I was another statistic, although without any hope of being tested, like anyone who has not had their coronavirus status confirmed, I wasn't even that.

I'm used to investigating outbreaks of disease in a population. It just happens that the populations I deal with are groups of sheep or cows rather than people and the diseases are species specific such as enzootic abortion or respiratory syncytial virus. Step one is always to confirm the diagnosis (using PCR tests to identify the pathogen or antibody tests to confirm exposure). Step two is to establish which animals have been exposed and infected. We do more tests, collect more facts, which is the basis of all medical practice, human or veterinary. From there, we can come up with a plan of control. How much simpler (and more effective) would it be to isolate those individuals infected, rather than isolate everyone? Without data, it is very hard to make a proper plan, let alone trust a computer-generated model.

But now, with my personal and presumed diagnosis, I had my own plans to make: how to survive a week without leaving the house or garden?

Life in a Time of Corona 4

I sat out my quarantine as per the instructions. My illness only lasted a couple of days. The sore throat gave way to a mild cough and I was quickly back to full health. I was in regular contact with all my colleagues via Skype, FaceTime and WhatsApp group chats, although I struggled to make the distorted image of my face that appeared on screen look any less ogre-some. Apparently, it's to do with the angle of the camera. Nobody I video-spoke with seemed too concerned though; they just seemed pleased to see me alive. I kept very busy. I listened to various online webinars about guidelines for the profession to follow during the crisis, addressing questions such as whether a fertility visit to see a herd of dairy cows was more or less crucial than the final part of a puppy's vaccination course, which would allow him to go for sanity-saving walks with his new owner. And how we could tackle either of these jobs while putting all concerned at the minimum risk. I could have sat an exam on the rules of furlough. This seemed like a new word, invented specifically to apply to the temporary laying-off of thousands of staff during this lockdown, but in fact it is an ancient word, dating back to the time of religious missionaries, who would be granted a leave of absence presumably after a tour of missioning duty. I bet lexicographers, accountants and HMRC officials never thought they'd be using this word so frequently. Mind you, a lot is happening at the moment that we would have never thought we'd be doing. Or not doing.

I counted down the days of isolation. Luckily, the greengrocer in Thirsk was happy to deliver. The box of fruit and vegetables was left at the gate. Were we eating more than usual, or was it just that the only source was the one fruit bowl? I read some books and did some writing. Luckily, I have a cycling machine in the garage. This gets a lot of use, during the long, cold winter months and the almost equally long weekends on call as I wait for my phone to ring. Once my fever had subsided, I felt fine and it was time to get back on the bike. Fortunately, the WiFi signal magically reaches as far as the garage, so the long sessions of sweating it out were made more tolerable by Netflix. The kids, like many millions of others across the world, were off school, so we all took turns on the exercise equipment. They had schoolwork emailed daily and set about it diligently. At least, being teenagers, they are reasonably self-sufficient and we haven't had to get too involved in actual teaching – I'm not sure how well that would go. The sun came out, so we set up the slack-line and the table-tennis table. Thank goodness for having a garden. I planned that we should watch some classic films, together as a family. *The Usual Suspects*, met with approval, but some of my other suggestions resulted in people drifting off to their bedrooms, with only the smallest attempt at an excuse. Film or no film, at least, the family is enjoying meal-time together. This only usually happens when we are away on holiday. Though this feels like anything but a holiday.

My sister dropped off some shopping. It was a long detour from Leeds, where she lives and I felt remiss not to have asked her in for coffee. She wouldn't have come in anyway – she dropped the bags off at the customary broom-length away and had a quick chat from the other side of the fence. I've ordered more food today from the greengrocers. At the bottom of the shopping list I wrote: *Good news! I'm out later this week!*

Life in a Time of Corona 5

Once my quarantine was over I could get back to work. The first early morning job of my first day back was to take the dog for a walk. Emmy has buckets full of energy and it's usually a challenge to get her lead on before leaving the house. She rushes with such speed. However, on that morning a lead wasn't necessary. The street was so empty that she had more chance of being struck by an asteroid than being hit by an oncoming car.

At the surgery, a skeleton staff had been holding the fort. Of course, all routine procedures had been put on hold. (For how long, I wondered? When restrictions are eventually lifted the amount of outstanding work will be a challenge to manage.)

But there was still plenty to do. My first job of the morning was to head straight out. A dairy herd needed a fertility visit. Instinctively, this does not sound like crucial work – the checking of cows for pregnancy and helping those with poor fertility to become pregnant. But this constitutes a vital part of the food chain and so falls into the category of *essential* work and made me a *keyworker*. For once, dairy farmers are being appreciated as "vital". As I headed out through yet more silent roads, I couldn't help but raise a wry smile. Not long ago, when milk products were being driven in from Eastern Europe by the tanker-load, British dairy farming was apparently held in low esteem. The tables have turned. The cows presented no coronavirus risk (although they can be affected by a different, bovine coronavirus; it doesn't cause panic and is usually very mild) and the farmer stood a healthy but unsociable distance away as I palpated ovaries and scanned one cow after another. Most of them were pregnant, ensuring a full lactation in due course. There were some calves to castrate and disbud too but this was impossible to do without close contact between vet and calf-holder, so had to be put off until safer times. Goodness knows how many of these jobs will have stacked up by later this year!

My next visit, also deemed *essential* by the powers that be, was to inspect and supervise the export of some cheese powder; it was destined for the opposite side of the world. I had to check the health provenance of the milk from which the cheese powder was derived, to make sure it wasn't carrying any diseases. It was hardly the cutting edge of clinical veterinary practice, but certification work like this is important to uphold food standards – a very important veterinary role, but one that fewer and fewer vets are qualified to undertake. The accreditation process has become laborious and convoluted. I usually have a visit like this every week or so and they need to continue despite "lockdown". On arrival, I did my best to maintain a safe distance, although the entry into the building – controlled by security key fob – could not be easily performed at broom's length.

Needless to say, the dairy-based-powder export was hassle-free and signatures and stamps were applied to all the documents as required. I'd done my part in facilitating international trade, deemed to be so essential. On the drive back to the practice, I pondered the rationale behind this and there seemed to be some glaring paradoxes. What I'd just done was not essential, far from it, but it was allowed as a means of keeping the economy moving. As I made my way up the empty high street in Boroughbridge, past the closed cafes and hairdressers with locked doors, it seemed to me that there was a much more pressing economy which needed to be supported – one much closer to home than where my cheese powder was destined.

Life in a Time of Corona 6

Over the last few weeks, a couple I know have evaded the lockdown and enjoyed a huge amount of freedom. Before you report them to the police for contravening the restrictions, the couple are rabbits, Luna and Boris. By night they sleep in a lovely, two-tiered hutch. By day, they frequent a huge, moveable run and an even more moveable Toblerone-shaped "pod", which are linked by a bendy, rabbit-sized tube. It is a superb arrangement for a pair of rabbits and they are very lucky. But the current COVID-19 clampdown, with most of the family at home, most of the time, has meant that they can be freed and can roam the garden for hours at a time, rather than just the occasional hour when they can be supervised at the weekend. It's been a miserable month, but Boris and Luna exploring the garden and binking in the sun has been a joy to watch.

Over the last few weeks, a couple I know have evaded the lockdown and enjoyed a huge amount of freedom. Before you report them to the police for contravening the restrictions, the couple are rabbits, Luna and Boris. By night they sleep in a lovely, two-tiered hutch. By day, they frequent a huge, moveable run and an even more moveable Toblerone-shaped "pod", which are linked by a bendy, rabbit-sized tube. It is a superb arrangement for a pair of rabbits and they are very lucky. But the current COVID-19 clampdown, with most of the family at home, most of the time, has meant that they can be freed and can roam the garden for hours at a time, rather than just the occasional hour when they can be supervised at the weekend. It's been a miserable month, but Boris and Luna exploring the garden and binking in the sun has been a joy to watch.

Last Sunday they were briefly confined back to barracks. It was time for mowing the lawn. I enjoy mowing the lawn, but it's usually a rushed job, squeezed in between others. Not now, though. To refill the petrol tank and crank the engine reminded me that spring was definitely here, that seasons change and that times move on. I was positively excited to be walking, with purpose, up and down the lawn again and again.

If it hadn't been the lawn, it would have been the garage doors, desperate for a coat of new paint. Countless families over the country must have been thinking the same thing: the garden fence, the shed or the garage doors need painting. Doubtless, some, in their lockdown boredom, would have also considered then watching that paint dry. But for this afternoon, I ignored the painting challenge and set about firing up the mower. For once, the task was pleasantly time-consuming, especially when I found huge tracts of previously undiscovered moss taking space where grass should have been. It's perfectly matched green was an excellent disguise but I knew it needed to come out, so I set about it with a rake, scarifying until I was covered with sweat. Yes, emergency veterinary work was busy, but the spare hours which would have been filled with gym, swim training, socializing, meeting people, being a human being could be diverted to my new task of moss removal.

If it hadn't been the lawn, it would have been the garage doors, desperate for a coat of new paint. Countless families over the country must have been thinking the same thing: the garden fence, the shed or the garage doors need painting. Doubtless, some, in their lockdown boredom, would have also considered then watching that paint dry. But for this afternoon, I ignored the painting challenge and set about firing up the mower. For once, the task was pleasantly time-consuming, especially when I found huge tracts of previously undiscovered moss taking space where grass should have been. Its perfectly matched green was an excellent disguise, but I knew it needed to come out, so I set about it with a rake, scarifying until I was covered with sweat. Yes, emergency veterinary work was busy, but the spare hours which would have been filled with gym, swim training, socialising, meeting people, being a human being, could be diverted to my new task of moss removal.

I felt lucky. I could rid any vexatious thoughts by scratching at the moss. There must be many people without moss, without even a garden or open space or access to fresh air. Is that a basic right we should have, Mr Hancock? And what if, confined to a small house and moss-free garden, we disagreed with our spouse. What if one half thinks, for example, that Mr Hancock and his team are doing a superb job, captaining a ship through torrid waters, while the other thinks the shortage of PPE for healthcare workers is an egregious crime or that the profound lack of testing for COVID-19 at the beginning has left the country hamstrung without data? There are sure to have been more inter-familial arguments over recent weeks because of the LOCKDOWN, and maybe some more serious than purely familial political disagreement. I really hope the protracted abolition of normal life has been worth it. For now, though, I was content that my lawn looked tidier. It was time to re-release the rabbits but, despite my moss-fuelled catharsis, I still had doubts and unanswered questions. The rabbits hopped out. Maybe I should ask Boris? He lolloped across the newly cut grass, ears bouncing. I doubted he could give me any answers.

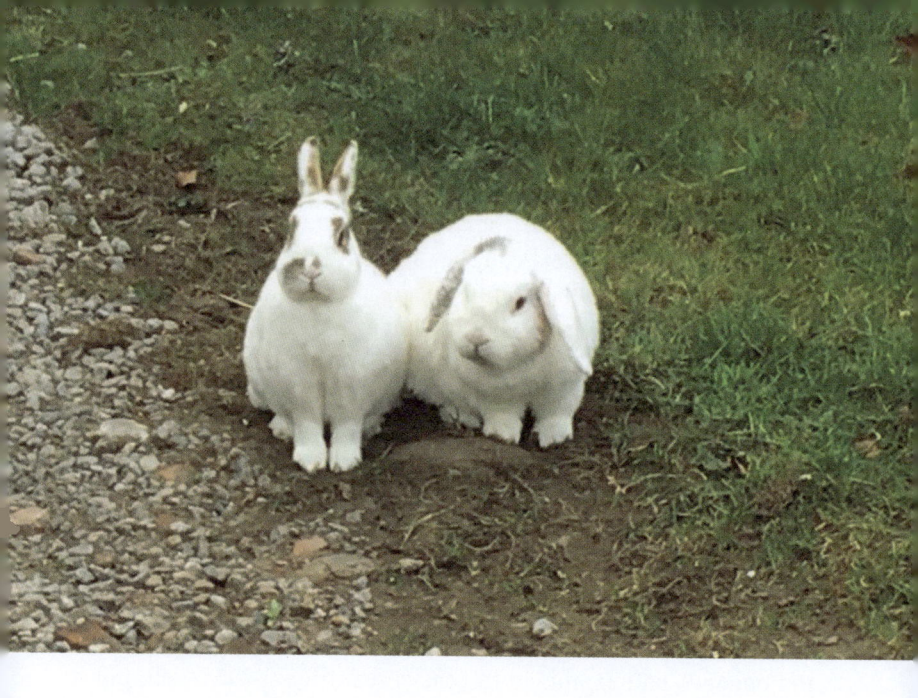

Spleen Out

We have been doing our best to triage cases over the phone, sometimes with the aid of emailed photographs or even videos. Some non-urgent cases can be successfully managed in this fashion, to minimise the number of people coming to the surgery. The veterinary governing bodies have allowed some laxity on the usually very strict guidelines about making a diagnosis and prescribing treatment, but it is far from ideal. The small abrasion on a cat's leg, for instance, was part of a bigger problem and not spotted by the owner or her camera. The fact that the cat was covered in multiple scabs as a result of an allergy was not apparent on the slightly blurred photo, nor did it become evident in the lengthy, lockdown induced phone discussion. The tube of topical cream that was prescribed was never going to be sufficient to treat the systemic problem. Luckily this became evident quite quickly, and once we had examined the cat in real life, all was well, but it highlighted the difficulty inherent in having to work out what to see and what to deal with remotely. A case of vomiting and diarrhoea is simple enough, but the dog who has vomited six times overnight certainly needs to be seen. Is it just a bad case of gastritis or is there a piece of corn-on-the-cob obstructing the bowel? A proper examination is essential, to palpate the abdomen and possibly followed up with X-rays. Trying to make these decisions by phone is a huge challenge.

One patient had me worried. Milo the terrier's clinical signs were non-specific. These are hard cases to manage even with the dog in front of you, let alone over the phone. The message suggested he was lying in odd places and didn't want to go upstairs. The signs were vague, but an owner who is concerned about a pet's unusual behaviour always flashes warning signs. After a brief telephone conversation, I knew I'd need to get hands-on with Milo. The terrier and his owner arrived at the practice very swiftly (given the quiet roads) and waited outside as instructed. I collected Milo via a lengthy lead and took him inside so I could examine him. On the surface he looked quite happy, but his body and legs were weak. Closer inspection revealed a few bigger problems. His gums were pale and, if a dog can have such a symptom, his face was sallow. There is a certain look worn by a sick dog and it's all about the eyes. It is as non-specific as lying in odd places and not wanting to go upstairs. I was immediately concerned.

Milo's abdomen was not as relaxed as it should have been. I examined this in more detail, balloting gently. Balloting has nothing to do with a secret voting system! It is the process of examining an abdomen by placing a hand on one side and tapping the other side with the other hand. If there is fluid in the abdomen, you can feel it vibrating as you tap. I could feel the characteristic "fluid thrill" as I did this to Milo. The next and quite simple job was to perform a peritoneal tap, which revealed that the aberrant fluid was blood, and an ultrasound scan confirmed that it was coming from a ruptured splenic tumour.

I stuck my head out of the practice door to explain to Milo's mum that he needed emergency surgery. It wasn't long before I'd removed Milo's cancerous spleen. His recovery was smooth and uneventful and, after a restful night on a drip, he went home the next day, very much brighter. It was a happy outcome and evidence enough that there is no substitute for a proper clinical examination. It is, after all, what is instilled into all vets from our very first day at Vet School.

New Life, Cicero and Tacitus

Is life getting back to normal? For some, maybe, but for most, no. Late one evening my phone pinged with a message. Attached to the message was a photograph. It was a picture of a nasty discharge from a llama's vulva. Aside from being something of a surprise, it was unlike anything I'd seen from the back of a llama before.

"And she's definitely not pregnant," came the corollary to the message. Whilst the image on my phone looked irregular, I felt able to provide some advice remotely, fulfilling (anti-)social-distancing regulations as required. It might be simply a vaginal infection, or worse an infection within the uterus – maybe endometritis. But it could be something more serious. I ran through the options in my head – was this a case that needed to be seen, or could it be managed "virtually"? I sent a message back suggesting a course of injections might work.

Inwardly, I suspected it would be better to examine the patient properly. After several emails and photos, I eventually had a telephone conversation and realised I'd need to compromise the anti-social distance rules to which the country was subjected in order to tend to a case of animal welfare. However, a llama's body is long, so the owner could hold the head end whilst I examined the rear and we would still be the crucial two metres apart.

I headed across the wild hills of Yorkshire, enjoying its empty roads. I listened to the radio for the latest news about what was happening in the world. Boris was out of hospital and busy quoting Cicero, the Roman statesman who gamely tried to uphold republican principles during various political crises in the establishment of the Roman Empire.

When I arrived on the farm it was clear that my patient did, as I had suspected, need more help than could be given by phone or email. I felt inside with my lubricated and gloved hand, not knowing quite what to expect. There were some solid bits inside the llama's vagina. I quickly ascertained that the solid bits were feet. The discharge was, contrary to the owner's previous assertion, due to a pregnancy, but an unexpected one and I needed to deliver a cria. A cria is the name for a baby alpaca or llama.

Llamas have very long necks and long legs, too, so a difficult birth is always challenging to sort out. In this case, the cria's neck was bent right back, it's head a long way in and hard to reach. After some work, I managed to get everything lined up and shortly the baby was delivered. Sadly, it was premature and dead. It had clearly died some time earlier and there was no way that the outcome could have been any better. Mum would be fine though. The baby was destined never to survive, but at least a healthy mum was a good outcome.

Everyone was disappointed, but pragmatic enough to know that we couldn't have done anything differently. On my way home, I switched the radio off, fed up with the diatribe from the media and government. I pondered the words of Cicero and his Roman colleagues and also the words of Tacitus, possibly the most renowned of all the Roman commentators. His most famous line referred to the governing bodies: "They make a desert and call it peace". As I traversed the empty roads of the Dales and headed through empty towns and villages on my way back to the surgery, I couldn't help but see what he meant – it certainly seemed like a desert.

Keeping Your Head

I've been trying to follow the advice in Kipling's famous poem "If" about keeping my head etc. Normally, I'm very good at this but the current restrictions and general lack of a proper plan is playing havoc with normality. Under normal circumstances, I'm good at assessing risk and mitigating its consequences by devising a practical solution. It's a self-protection mechanism, which vets have to acquire from their very first day. One cow I treated this week had a huge swelling in front of her udder. As I arranged her, with the farmer safely standing two metres away, so I could insert a long, thick and sharp needle into said lump to ascertain its contents, memories came flooding back of the first time I carried out this procedure. It was in my first weeks of veterinary practice, when I was at the bottom of an exponential learning curve of risk and consequence. Several minutes after inserting the needle, with stars spinning in front of my eyes, I picked myself up from the pile of straw, some five metres way from the patient, into which I had been kicked. But it was a lesson quickly learnt and this week's bovine needle aspirate, despite rapid-fire feet, was accomplished without catastrophe.

But rhetoric of catastrophe is the order of the day. Whilst commenting on the possibility of the long-awaited return to school for our children, a friend was concerned. "It's a matter of life and death though, isn't it?" she said. But is it? At the time of writing and according to the Office of National Statistics, of seven million children in the UK between five and fourteen years, only one has died as a result of the coronavirus outbreak. Phrases like a "second wave" and "spike" immediately invoke fear. Would the nation feel less anxious if words like "ripple" or "blip" were used? Or maybe "bleb"?

We are doing our best to avoid a second bleb by fastidiously following the rules or guidelines, some of which offer more practical solutions to mitigate risks than others. The new plastic screen in the waiting room, for example, will surely offer a good level of protection for client-facing staff. Before I headed out to calve a heifer, I briefly looked at some of the other directives we had recently received. If we couldn't stand two metres apart, we should position ourselves "back to back" where possible!

I was still pondering how that would work when I arrived at the farm, to see the young heifer in question charging around the dimly lit pen. She had two large feet sticking out of her back end. The wildness in her eyes told me that this would be another exercise in risk assessment. Proper practical measures would be required to mitigate the very real risk of catastrophe. Eventually, after several abortive attempts, my patient was captured. It didn't take long to realise that a caesarean section was needed. Despite instilling plenty of local anaesthetic to numb her side, for the second time in one morning I was dodging lightning-fast kicks, while trying not to incise my own hands with my scalpel. As the youngster objected to my efforts, the job was made even more difficult as she contracted her abdominal muscles, forcing part of her swollen rumen out of the hole I'd just made. This bleb was the size of a space-hopper and I even found myself using my forehead to try and keep it in place. Eventually, despite huge challenges, as always, it was done. Assisted by the farmer pulling on one leg, a huge calf was delivered onto the straw. The new mum, now calm, looked on. I pondered my flagrant disregard for the guidance of "working back to back". But, like I say, vets are good at finding practical solutions to risky situations.

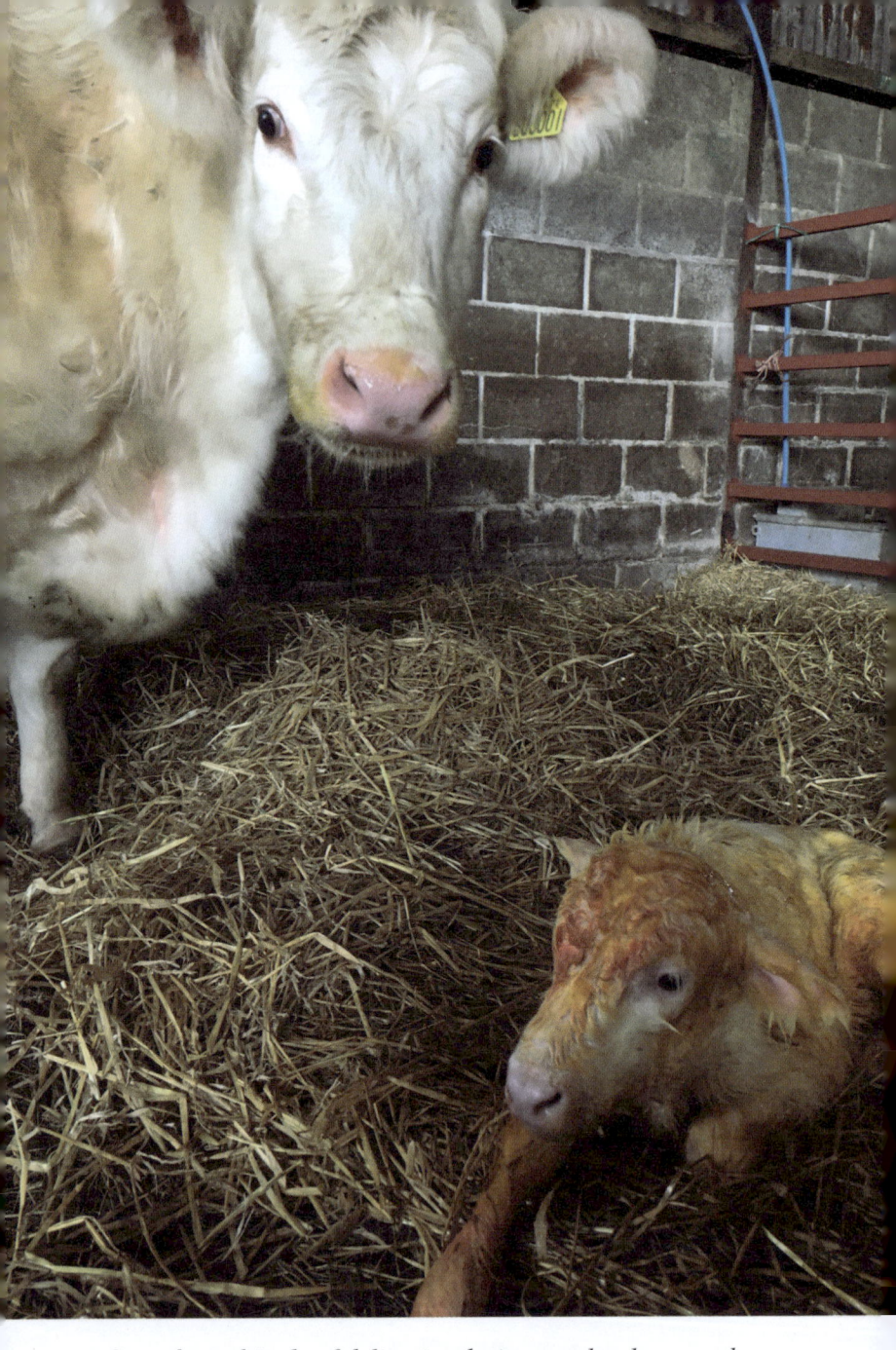

One of a multitude of deliveries during another busy week.

Life in a Time of Corona 7

Everyone must surely agree that it's good to be able to get out and about; that everyone can at long last enjoy the beautiful countryside, fresh air and wonderful weather again. But back in the middle of the corona clampdown, tension was palpably rising. Concern over health, job security, the sanity of our family and friends, and the stress of the restrictions, all played a part. I felt fortunate, because work allowed me to get out as we still had farm animals to look after. Others were less fortunate. I couldn't begin to imagine how hard it was for those with no access to the outside, like the residents of the small terraced house just along the street from where we live, no bigger than two up and two down and without any sign of a garden or yard. The child's colourful picture of a rainbow in the window showed support for the health workers. I felt for the family – especially the child – suffering without a garden to escape into. How people in those countries with much more draconian lockdowns have coped I don't know. I heard a radio report describing how in Italy, one family with two children had literally not left the house for six weeks. The problems this brings are profound, and the mother described how it was a case of "getting through" each day.

It is a busy time of year for vets and farmers and after a week with calvings too numerous to recount, a multitude of lambings and associated veterinary emergencies, I reflected on the nature of this work. Few of the procedures would have been possible had I stuck rigidly to the two-metre rule, but each case was a matter of clinical judgement and assessment of the risk both to myself and the client. Trying to find ways to manage each situation to keep ourselves safe while ensuring the animal was treated appropriately and did not suffer was a challenge. After work, I was glad to get my quotient of exercise and one sunny afternoon I jumped on my bike to enjoy an hour or so of solitude. Everywhere was, as expected, very quiet – the roads were like being back in the fifties, apparently.

I overtook a couple of cyclists, at high speed and with a wide berth and soon I came across a farmer who had been tending his sheep. I watched his sturdy lambs in the field on the left, thriving on the new grass and skipping and playing with their friends in the warm spring sunshine. After a torrid and waterlogged end to winter, and despite all the chaos, lambing time could not have been better. I expected the farmer, who was about to climb into a bright yellow Land Rover, must be full of the joys of spring. It was a wonderful day, his stock looked wonderful and his job – out in the fresh air of North Yorkshire – had hardly been hindered at all by COVID.

He stepped purposefully into my two-metre space from the side of the road, standing on the verge as I toiled up the incline. "We've had too many [swear word] cyclists like you!" he bellowed, with more aggression than I'd encountered anywhere. I looked ahead at the open road, and then behind to check I wasn't about to be swallowed up by a huge peloton. Both were empty.

Maybe the farmer had a deep hatred of cyclists? Maybe he simply had a deep hatred of people? Maybe he was just hassled, stressed and fretting about the restriction of normal life by COVID? If so, I have to say, with acres of his own farm land to enjoy and fresh air in abundance, he was in a much better position than most. If you're reading this piece, yellow Land Rover-driving sheep farmer, I hope you're feeling more relaxed now.

Prolapses Two Times and Scooby the World's Most Unlucky Cat

Emergencies have taken up much of my veterinary time recently. This isn't just because the reduced number of routine jobs has left a predominance of urgent work. I seem to have been rushing from pillar to post more than usual.

One of the most urgent cases presented a week or so ago. An alpaca had given birth and, immediately afterwards, the whole uterus was pushed out. This is called a uterine prolapse and is a serious event for any animal. For a sensitive soul like an alpaca, it's an urgent matter of life and death. I dropped everything and rushed to the farm as quickly as the speed limit would allow. Mum was surprisingly alert given the fact that the bright red, rugby-ball-sized uterus was dangling out of her vulva. Whilst this is a reasonably common problem in sheep and cows, it was only the second I'd treated in a camelid. However, the process of repair is the same, except for the fact that in this species everything seems to be much more delicate. Despite being a relative novice at replacing an alpaca's insides, everything went remarkably smoothly and the awful sight was soon corrected.

A few nights later, at the unsavoury hour of half past one in the morning, I found myself replacing another prolapse, this time in (or actually more accurately, out of) a cow. But it didn't start like that. It started as a calving. A very difficult calving. After much effort, the monstrous calf eventually slid with a plop onto the straw. Under the lights of the tractor, the farmer, his wife and I grinned with satisfaction, happy to have solved the problem so far. I stood up to stretch my aching back. As I rocked forwards, I could only groan again as the sack-of-potatoes-sized uterus slid out, in one smooth, flowing movement, with considerably more ease than the oversized calf had done just moments earlier. My night's work was not over! In fact, the hard part was just about to start. It reminded me of a terribly long evening's work, many years ago, which started with a cow that had inadvertently spiked itself on a long metal rod. It had penetrated all the way into her chest cavity and this necessitated a lengthy suturing job. Just as this was completed, she started to calve. After some manipulation and pulling, we got the calf out, only for her to push out her uterus too. I finally managed to replace the uterus as the cow gasped her last breath and expired. Luckily, this week's case didn't do this and has hopefully gone on to raise her giant calf.

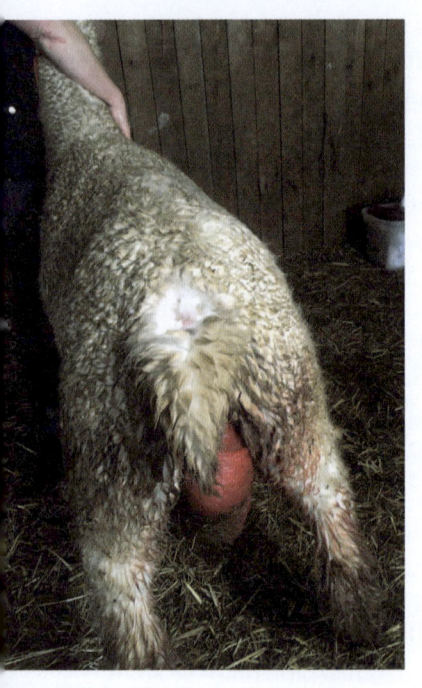

A few more days passed and I added a sheep to my weekly prolapse collection, but this one was simple – just the size of a tennis ball – during daytime hours and without any panic. The farmer brought it to see me at the practice. An epidural, a good clean and gentle but firm pressure was all that was required to pop it back in, followed by a special suture to keep it all neatly in place. Just like a Christmas present.

My final emergency was Scooby. He was possibly the unluckiest cat in recent times. During a period when the roads of North Yorkshire have been quieter than any of us can remember, Scooby had been so remarkably unlucky as to have been hit by one of the very few cars around. He was the only cat we had seen involved in a road traffic collision since lockdown, but his injuries proved to be extensive. His right hind leg was floppy and painful and my X-rays revealed multiple fractures to his tibia. His injuries would present an altogether different problem from the miscellaneous uterine issues at the start of the week.

The Dog that Said 'Hello'

For a few reasons, I've been thinking about talking dogs recently. A friend, who lives just down the road, happened to pass our house one evening this week. We had not seen her for a while, through a combination of COVID restrictions and her elderly dog having recently been put to sleep just a few months earlier. We didn't even come across each other on dog walks anymore. But she had a new dog on trial and he was pulling her along the road. I spotted her from the sitting room window, waved and rushed to the front door to catch up and have a chat.

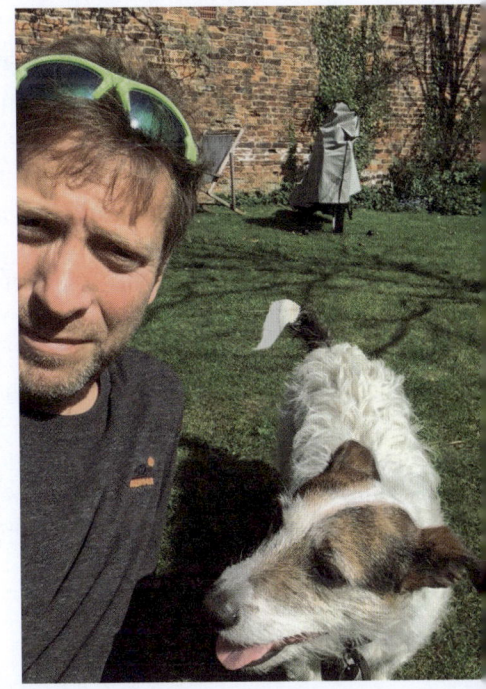

Jake the Staffie was a rescue dog, as all Lindsey's dogs had been over the years. Kind and caring and devoted to her dogs, Lindsey was missing a canine companion, especially during the restrictions. She had agreed to take Jake for a week to see if they were right for one another and this was the first time she'd taken him for a walk. From the doorstep, Anne and I could catch up and meet the new dog from a safe distance. We naturally assumed positions as if we were the apices of an isosceles triangle. A sunny evening, with no beeper in my pocket and whilst catching up with an old friend, was a perfect excuse to open a bottle of wine. Everyone was fraught under the current circumstances and this impromptu and al fresco rendezvous was a welcome relief. Conversation immediately turned to Jake. The oversized Staffie's tail wagged constantly and his open mouth wore a huge grin all the time. He was certainly endearing, but the most amusing thing about him were the talking noises he made all the time, as if trying to join in the conversation.

Jake's conversational skills were undoubtedly impressive and reminded me of a recent episode when I'd, inexplicably, been fast asleep on the sofa one Saturday afternoon. This occurrence is sufficiently rare to put it on a par with a lunar eclipse or other unusual celestial event, but fatigue had obviously caught up with me. I'd apparently been asleep for an hour or more and I was bleary and confused when the dog wandered in and vigorously licked every part of my sleeping face that was poking out above the woolly blanket that was keeping me warm. Emmy, the dog, who was as surprised as I was to find me reclined and inert in the daytime, then stretched and said "Hello," in a matter-of-fact kind of way.

At least, I am fairly certain that she said "hello". I called Anne to confirm the miracle. Emmy is very capable, but nobody had ever heard her talk before.

"The dog has just said 'hello'!" I shouted, through a soporific haze, which was sufficient to confirm that it was some sort of hallucination or sleep-induced mistake on my part.

There are many other special skills that dogs have, some beyond the comprehension of us mere humans. Recent research suggests that some dogs have the capability to sniff out certain types of cancer; some dogs can sense the onset of an epileptic seizure and I've heard various stories of dogs that predict the onset of seismic activity. There is certainly a spectrum of canine sensory ability that transcends the human senses, some of which we are, no doubt, still to learn. I looked at Emmy that sleepy afternoon, convinced she was about to launch into a full sentence. But Jake the stocky Staffie, on the sunny evening this week, did not exactly look like he was about to recite a Shakespearean sonnet. That said, he was considerably more verbose than the terrier on Esther Rantzen in the 1980s which, with such clarity, could only say "sausages"!

Butcher's Dog

There is a butcher in Richmond who reads the Country Week section of *The Yorkshire Post*. There are probably many butchers in Richmond who read this newspaper, but I know for certain that there is at least one, because he keeps sending his dog-owning customers to see me. I've had a steady stream of lame dogs arrive at the surgery because of his (possibly unfounded) recommendation. This is very kind and generous, because writing this column doesn't confer upon me any extra veterinary capability to fix a spaniel with a sore leg. That takes the phrase "omni-competent" to a new level.

Once upon a time, all vets were required to be exactly that: omni-competent. It was expected that a newly qualified vet would (and should) be competent in all aspects of veterinary practice, right from day one! This is a tall order, but one which we seemed to consider eminently achievable as my cohort of vets emerged, white-coated, from vet school into the world of clinical practice. Some days, in the true spirit of omni-competency, instead of being white-coated, we'd actually be brown-coated because, even in the 1990s, some vets still wore a long, brown coat to do farm work, while white was reserved for small animal duties. Apart from having useful pockets for putting thermometers, stethoscopes, bottles and syringes, a long brown cotton coat was not a very practical outfit on a farm. My brown coat quickly gave way to a plastic waterproof, which afforded superior Personal Protective Effect.

In these post-brown coat days of veterinary medicine, omni-competency represents an even bigger challenge, especially for our new vets. As client expectation has risen, in part because diagnostic and surgical opportunities have expanded, there is more pressure upon vets to get a rapid and firm diagnosis and offer specialist surgical solutions. At one time, the constantly sneezing cat, for example, would eventually be admitted for an anaesthetic so that the back of its nasopharynx could be examined to check for the unwelcome presence of a *nasopharyngeal polyp*. An eagle-eyed young vet would spot the pea-sized nobble, grab it with forceps and pull it out, effecting an immediate cure. Nowadays, it is the magic of the CT scanner, which has eagle eyes of its own, that takes over responsibility for finding the troublesome polyp.

It's the same with a lame horse. Anything more than a simple case of pus-in-the-foot tends to send owners running to see a horse specialist, who spends his days exploring the nuances of an equine lameness. This is a good thing, but it leaves the neophyte vet missing another important opportunity to make his or her own diagnosis and learn from it. Omni-competency is not so easy now, which makes it vital that the more senior members of the profession assist, encourage and advise the new members, to help them along this rocky road. Recently, I had a great opportunity to do just that. Afternoon surgery had just finished and an emergency call to calve a cow came in. It was an ideal opportunity for Molly, our recently graduated vet, to do her first calving.

"Do you want to come along, Molly? I'll go first and you follow on," I suggested and her eyes lit up with an enthusiasm which had been building during her five years at vet school. An enthusiasm which I remembered well. On the farm, I stood back and let Molly take the lead, talking her through the various stages, offering guidance where needed. The calving was a squeeze, but not too tricky and this had been a perfect first case for her to learn. She did a great job and, from what I can see, the next generation of omni-competent vets is shaping up very nicely indeed!

Opposite: Molly's first delivery.

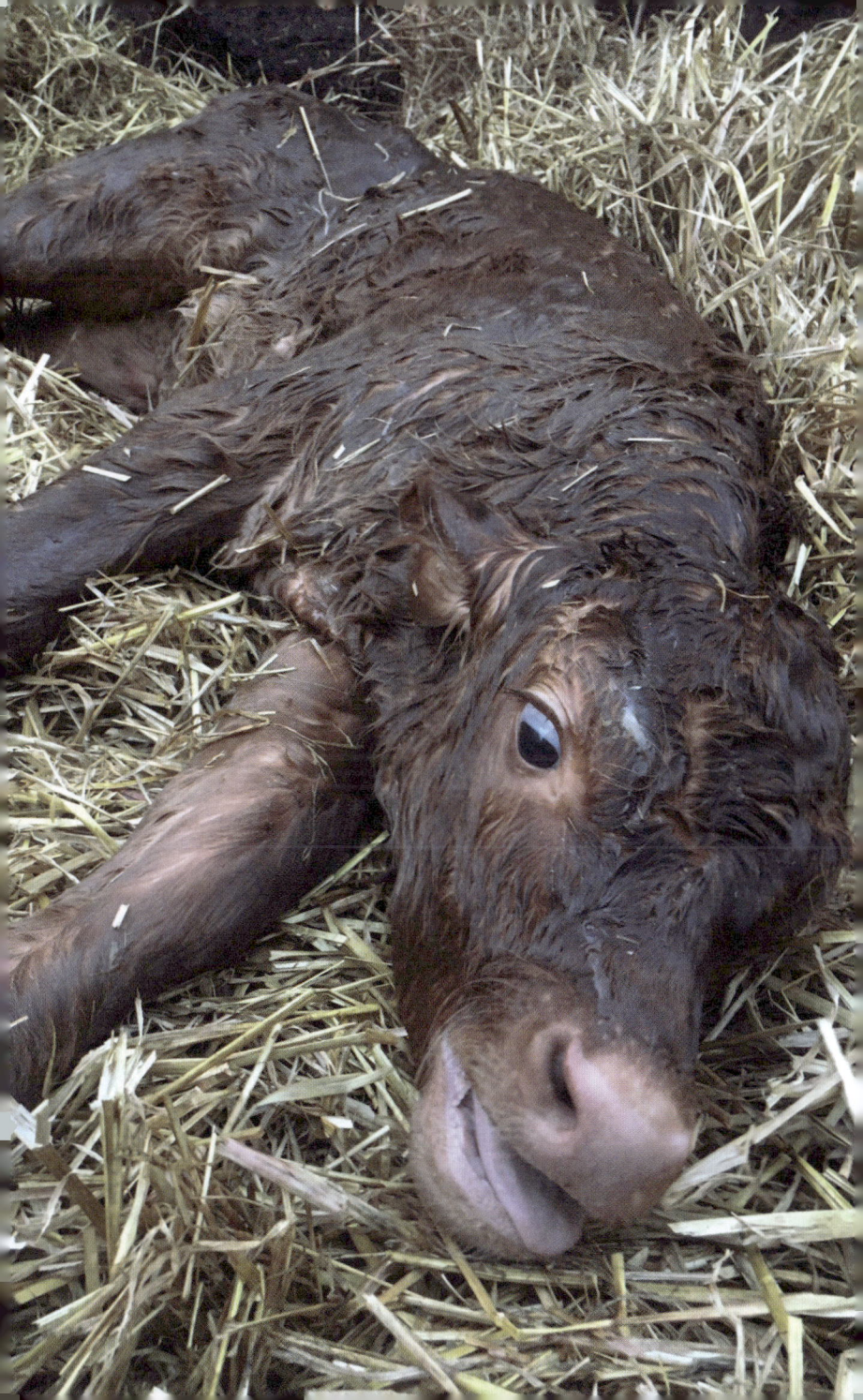

Minty Gloves

Vets are experts when it comes to gloves. We wear standard latex ones when inserting fingers up dogs' bottoms to express the contents of their anal glands or to palpate the prostate. I wear them when on a farm, mainly to reduce the likelihood of getting pathogens on my hands, which might be hard to scrub off, no matter how many times I sing "happy birthday" to myself. We wear sterile surgical ones when in theatre. Some of us also wear amazingly long ones, which extend to the shoulder. These are required when the whole arm is inserted inside a cow, an important job to check the internal organs. These special, lengthy ones are called "rectal gloves", for obvious reasons. The best ones have a loop for putting your head through, to stop the glove slipping down past the elbow. It is the rectal glove equivalent of a set of braces.

Rectal gloves also come in a version called "extra sensitive", which can be useful when extra rectal sensitivity is required. But whatever the sensitivity, I also make sure I have plenty in my car boot. Running out of either type of glove – be it standard sized and latex or shoulder length and plastic – does not bear thinking about.

Because of recent viral problems, there is no doubt that many more people will have become experts in protective gloves, some wearing them everywhere they go. I've seen some people even wearing them whilst driving alone in their car! I suspect the suppliers of latex gloves must have struggled to keep up with the new, huge demand, extending as it has beyond the usual vets, dentists, medics and people who spray cars for a living. The reason I suspect this, is because one of the versions that arrived at the practice recently looked distinctly unconventional. I eyed them up with suspicion, because on the front of the box it said *Premium Grip Mint*. These were undeniably a niche product in the field of latex gloves. I'd never come across latex gloves with extra special grip as a benefit. And they were minty green, too!

I didn't have to wait long to investigate, because I had another set of anal glands to express. I removed one from the box, with its beautiful calligraphic writing, and pulled it on with a satisfying twang. The twang was quickly followed by an obvious minty-fresh smell and I realised that the deluxe gloves were not just minty in colour, but also in aroma. I wiggled my fingers and sniffed. These were certainly special gloves, and ones which the veterinary wholesaler must have had left on the shelf. The current short supply and high demand, I surmised, was a great opportunity to offload some unnecessarily fancy and usually unwanted gloves. I stroked my gloved palm and fingers to try to get a sense of the purported premium grip. There was, indeed, a subtle ribbing, but it was not possible to tell at this point whether the grip was actually premium. It was ironic that usually when a vet dons a latex glove, the very next application is one of gloopy lubricant, with the exact purpose of *reducing* grip. I was certain that my patient Wilbur, a Westie with bulging anal glands, would appreciate lubrication and a *lack* of grip. As I sniffed my gloved fingers, which smelt like toothpaste, one more time I couldn't help but wonder whether the inside of Wilbur's rectum would benefit from the same minty freshness. It reminded me of the first time I ever tried a funky new shower gel, which was liberally laced with tea tree and mint. That didn't go particularly well, as I recall! I watched for a surprised expression on Wilbur's face . . .

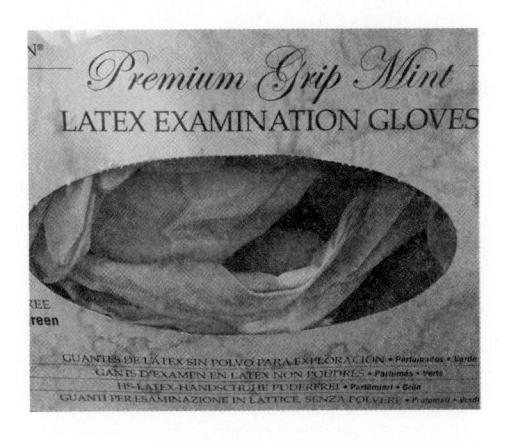

Zoomed Out

It's not that I'm a Luddite. Generally, I love technological advances, provided that they are just that – advances. At the moment, though, I am "Zoomed out". This sounds like a phrase from the vocabulary of a cameraman, applicable when nobody wants a close-up. I definitely feel a bit like that on a regular basis, but in this context what I mean is that I am getting fed up with virtual meetings. I know they have been a necessity over recent months, to facilitate both important meetings and vital yoga classes, but personally I'm struggling with them.

There is no doubt that these technologies have been essential in the battle to continue work in the face of social distancing. The emailed pictures of a dog's ear or sore foot have enabled treatment to be provided without a trip to the surgery, although the quality of the pictures seems to vary wildly, sometimes they are so pixelated that the images more closely resemble the Minecraft version of a dog (something I witness every time I poke my head into my youngest son's bedroom to check on his "home-schooling").

I had a great Zoom meeting with some Cambridge vet students recently. Some of them had missed out on their graduation ceremony on the lawns in front of the Vet School. I can still remember every minute of that amazing day, twenty-four years ago, almost to the day and I feel so sad for them, missing this culmination of all their hard work.

Practice Zoom meetings are of varying success due to lack of adequate broadband in parts of North Yorkshire and the vagaries of being on call. There is the perennial "it's the button at the bottom left" conflab when people can be seen but not heard. It is a button I find increasingly useful to deploy.

My Zoom experience reached its peak this week, however, when I had an interview with the Royal Television Society, to talk about my experiences over recent years in front of the camera. My venue of choice for the meeting, in the absence of a study crammed with classic literature, was the spare bedroom. We chatted for the customary forty minutes' worth of free Zoom time about the trials, tribulations and adventures I had enjoyed in the world of telly, all of which were unexpected.

It was only as the Zoom interview – destined for high-powered telly types to peruse online somewhere and sometime – drew to a close, that something caught my eye on the screen of my laptop. It was a huge, smiling, cuddly toy, won by my father in the kids' primary school summer fair many years ago. He was called Dodger and he was a bear. His benign grin made it hard to send him to the charity shop and his presence went unnoticed for most of the year. But this evening, as I'd tried my best to be sensible and erudite for the higher echelons of the RTS, Dodger's presence, sitting behind me in a rocking chair, undermined my efforts. I signed off and said my goodbyes, thankful that most of the work of a vet must be done actually rather than virtually. Animals have never heard of Zoom.

I met a new patient the following day, whose owner had been waiting patiently for such time as the new kitten could have her vaccinations. I peered into the cat box, before taking the fuzzy ball of fluff into the surgery.

"We couldn't think of what to call her," her owner explained. "Then it hit us: she's so fast and what with all these virtual meetings, we've decided to call her Zoom!"

Zoom the kitten.

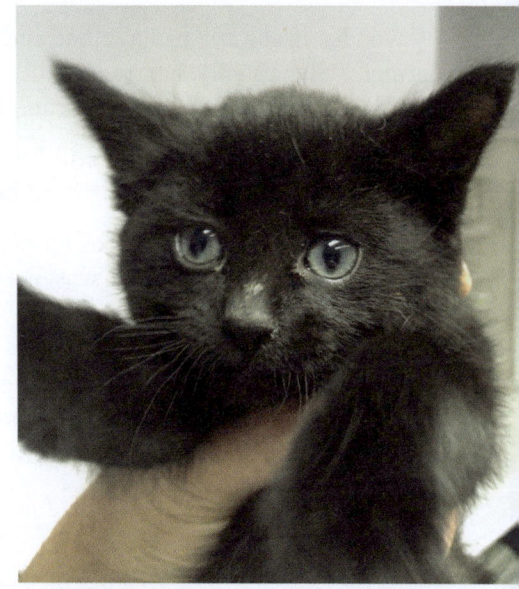

Pulling Feet

It was another Sunday afternoon calving and I arrived in Knaresborough to rapturous applause. I knew from previous experience that this was a very friendly town, having spent many a New Year in the pubs around the square. In fact, having enjoyed New Year's Eve celebrations in several other North Yorkshire towns, I can confirm that Knaresborough is certainly the friendliest of them all.

At first, I couldn't understand the excitement. Surely the whole town could not have been so delighted that the vet had arrived? I greeted the anxious farmer, saying, "I can't believe it. I've only just arrived and the whole town is clapping!"

"Oh, I think it's a 'clap for the NHS' event," he replied, at which point I remembered it was the celebration of seventy-two years of the Health Service. "Anyway, I'm glad you're here because we're really worried."

The cow in question was giving birth, but no proper progress had been made. Confusingly, there appeared to be some afterbirth hanging from her vulva beside an intact water bag.

"I wonder if she might have had one calf already?" queried the farmer. "She usually has twins, this old girl, but we've looked everywhere around the field and can't find a calf."

"Well don't worry," I reassured. "I'll be able to tell you exactly what is going on shortly. Can we get her in a crush?"

I cleaned my arms and applied lubricant as usual, but what I felt upon starting my examination was most unusual and not something I can recall ever having felt inside a cow before. There was no head, but there were some feet, upside down. Each foot was attached to a hock, which meant they were back feet. A calf coming backwards is a common cause of difficulty. But as I explored further, I found not two, but four back feet! With difficulty, I could pull all four of them into view, but it wasn't easy to identify which made a pair. It looked like a party was going on in there! Each foot was approximately the same size and all were exactly the same conker colour, so at first attempt it was impossible to match them up. In lambs, it's possible to feel far enough inside to work out which leg goes with which, but in this case, there was no space for me to reach past the jumble of feet. I would have to make an educated guess. I put my yellow calving rope on the first leg and my green rope on another. I pulled hard, but nothing budged, leading me to conclude that yellow and green ropes were not attached to the same calf. I tried again with another rope – this time blue. Would the yellow and blue combo work? I tried to calculate the statistics of guessing the correct combination. I thought this must definitely be right, but still no joy. I then attached my red rope to the fourth leg and pulled along with the yellow. It was third time lucky. After pushing the blue- and green-roped legs back in, the first calf, with red and yellow ropes on its legs, slid out with relative ease. For a twin, it was large and I relaxed a bit, because I knew that the hardest part was done. Another pull and calf number two, with blue and green ropes, emerged into the world, landing next to its twin. Everyone was relieved, because this had been a tense and challenging calving.

"Thank you very much. Your efforts have made an old farmer very pleased," were the parting words of thanks. He was so grateful, I half expected he was going to start clapping.

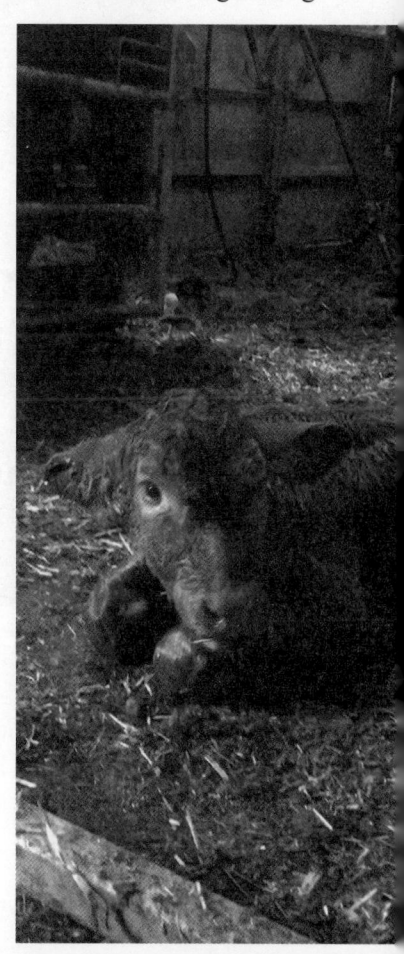

Pigs

Over the last few weeks, I've been lucky enough to treat a few pigs. Years ago, vets in general practice would regularly see a poorly pig and every farm had a few sows. There is an old day book at the practice, which records, in scrawled handwriting on faded paper, a visit all the way to Brough on the edge of the Westmorland plateau, to treat a pig with a skin condition, for which it received a bottle of lotion. In those days, a pig was treated as an individual. Modern pig practice is very different and modern pig farming seems to encourage the very opposite. The unit is managed as exactly that – a unit. For lots of reasons, a pig farmer now would never call a vet to see an individual with sores on its skin. In part, this is because the number of veterinary practices that specialise in pigs can be counted on the finger of two hands. Vets in those practices travel huge distances to oversee the health, welfare and performance of the animals under their care, but both the economics and the practicalities do not allow individual patient care for most.

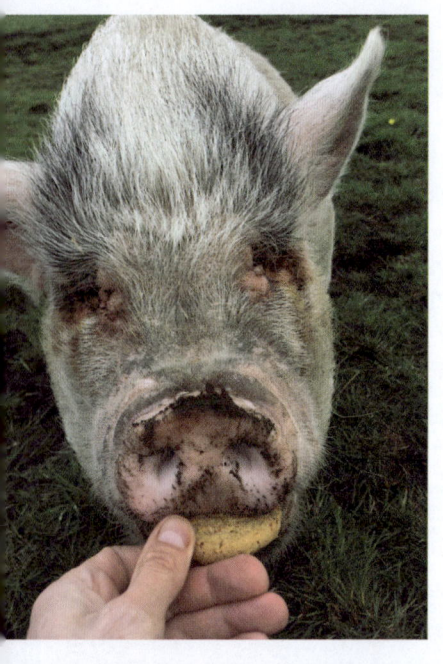

This is why I was glad to have been able to see several pigs. Even though an individual pig is hard to catch and manage, a pig is usually a pleasure to treat. The first pig was lame, with a swollen festering foot, unresponsive to the usual treatment. The farmer wanted the view of an expert, but today, I would have to do. From a distance, I could offer some advice and encouragement. The powers of healing are strong, especially when

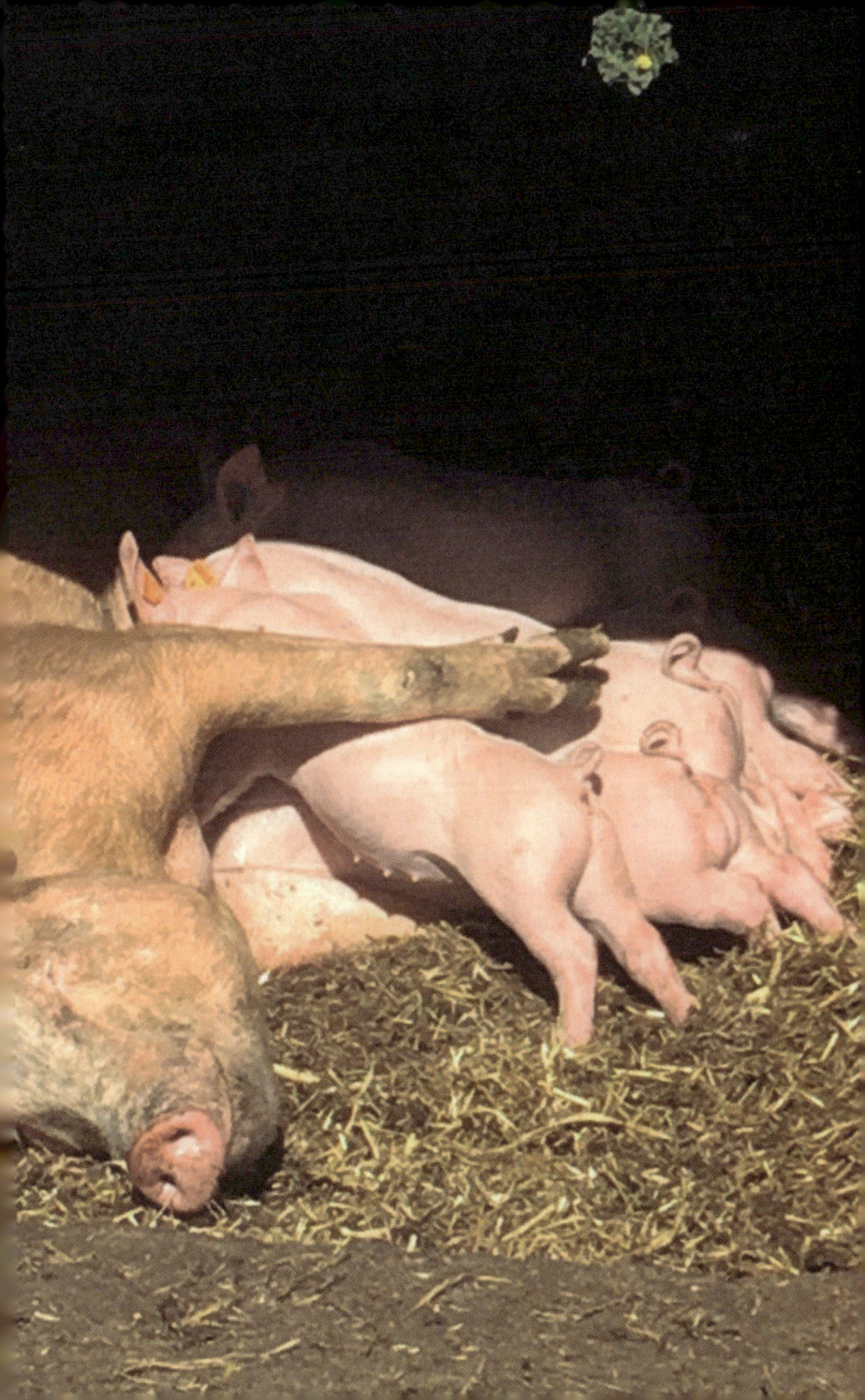

combined with the power of antibiotics. I dispensed a bottle and we hoped for the best. The sow had a litter to rear and so the alternative – premature slaughter – did not bear thinking about.

Pig two was an old friend and had no purpose for breeding or production of any kind. Gilbert was a micro-pig. At least, once he was a micro-pig. As "micro" pigs are prone to do, Gilbert continued to grow until he had attained the proportions of a normal sized pig. This was, in part, because his owner fed him on treats in addition to his normal piggy diet. Ice cream when it was hot, biscuits at other times. He also enjoyed his paddling pool and even had a teddy bear in his sty for company. Fortunately, Gilbert needed no treatment – he was a casual bystander as I sedated his best friend, a one tonne Clydesdale horse called Harvey. The only treatment Gilbert needed was a ginger biscuit, which he devoured greedily.

Pig three, Elsie, was more confusing, as she had suddenly refused to eat. With no other obvious signs to report, I knew this little piggy would prove to be a diagnostic challenge. I quizzed the owner about her habits and patterns of behaviour, but yielded no proper clues. Catching the patient so that I could examine her was also easier said than done. Of course, what every vet hopes for is a sky-high temperature, or some other clear sign of illness, offering an easy path to a cure, but Elsie had a normal temperature. Coupled with normal sounding heart and lungs, perfectly formed faeces, normal, healthy skin and a sound udder, I was struggling for a diagnosis. Could she have been stung in the mouth by a bee? I opted for a speculative injection, which I hoped would help. As I drove off, still scratching my head, I couldn't help thinking that I might need to draft in an actual pig expert. But a phone call the next day confirmed that, happily, Elsie was well and truly on the mend and her greedy-as-a-pig appetite was back to normal. This was great news, but left me not much the wiser!

Fleeced

The last few months have seen most of us trying out new tasks. Huge swathes of Britain have, inexplicably, turned their hands to the making of sourdough, like nascent bakers in the making. And we have all surely had a go at taming the flowing locks of our family by snipping in a more or less haphazard fashion in an attempt at a haircut. Judging by the chaos on the heads of many, hairdressers are certain to boom again once life returns to normal.

But this week, it was not snipping hair, nor baking bread which was my challenge. I was heading down the A1 to learn how to shear a sheep! Elizabeth, aka *The Wild Wool Shepherdess*, was my mentor and tutor for the day. She introduced me to her flock, which consisted of primitive breeds based on Icelandic and Shetland cross ewes. Whilst these traditional breeds would not win any prizes in the butchers' shops, it is for their wool that Elizabeth keeps them. It was lovely to meet a farmer with a passion for the old-fashioned ways. Elizabeth shears her sheep and makes rugs and felted products from their lustrous fleeces. Of course, on this traditional farm, there was never going to be noisy and hectic mechanical clippers. We each grabbed our handheld shears and picked a couple of ewes who were most in need of a trim. I watched and learned as Elizabeth snipped, following the contours of her ewe and readjusting her feet to support the sheep. She hadn't broken any records for speed, but that was not the point. We could hear the birds singing and feel the muscles and sinews of the sheep relax as the thick, lanolin-rich fleeces fell away in smooth, clean waves. Before long, it was my turn and I took a deep breath before making the first snip. Of course, the blades were sharp and pointy and one false move could lead to disaster. With the sheep sitting comfortably, I began. The outside of the back-left leg was first and I remembered the instruction to pull the skin taut to define the junction between sheep and fleece. I was soon in my stride and the process turned out to be easier than I'd imagined. Much like unpeeling a satsuma, there was a natural line to slice through, from which the fleece fell out and away from the sheep. The rhythmic sound of the shears was pleasantly relaxing. Just as pleasing was the production of a fully intact fleece lying on the grass and an unscathed sheep, considerably smaller than she'd been ten minutes before. Her flock-mates looked confused (if that's possible for a sheep) as I put her back in the pen, as if she was a newcomer. Maybe that would be the same response I'd get upon returning to work after my long-awaited haircut!

After a quick sandwich for lunch, it was time to turn the fleece into a rug! This process involved applying more wool to the back of the fleece and rubbing it with warm water and soap to allow the woolly fibres to interlock, forming a felt backing. It was the same process used one thousand years ago by the ancient settlers of Asia and the rampaging Mongols as they conquered land and sheltered in tents made of the same felt. It struck me that the success of those ancient civilisations must have been due to the sheep they tendered to and the versatile, warm and waterproof wool they produced.

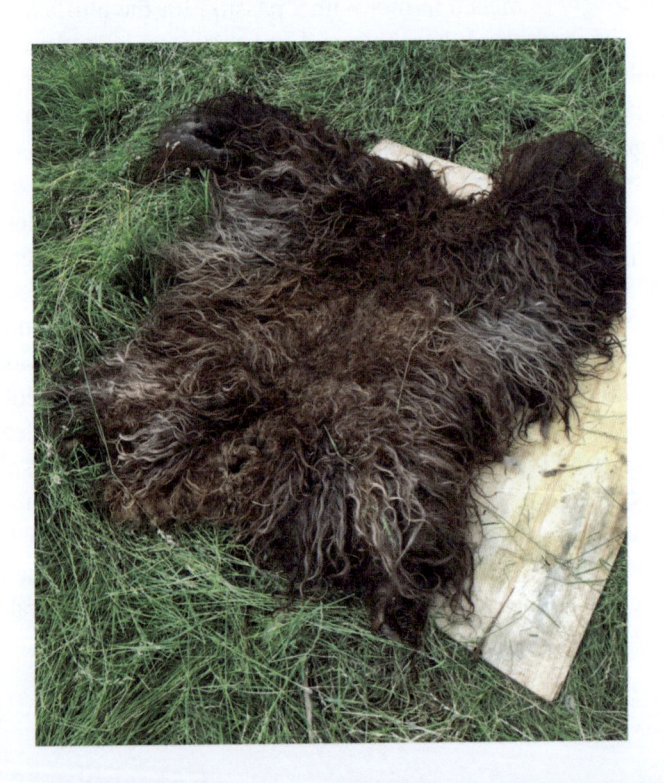

Baby Ferrets and Cria Kindergarten

One of the best things about being a vet is getting to meet so many baby animals. Even though we've seen thousands of kittens or puppies over the course of a career, it's still life-affirming on a daily basis. Luckily, on a difficult day, when the stresses and strains and the constant demands seem overwhelming, a cute puppy usually comes along at just the right moment to lift everyone's spirits. I remember one terrible day when a young Labrador belonging to a practice nurse had to be euthanised because of an inoperable tumour. Everyone was devastated, but there was no time to dwell on sad thoughts because the very next surgical case was a whelping bitch who needed a caesarean. The sadness was at least in some part washed away by the twelve bundles of squeaking fluff which had been brought into the world, completing yet another circle of life.

Recently, there seems to have been new life aplenty. A friend messaged me to see if I could help rehome some unexpected baby ferrets. Baby ferrets are called kits and I think the expectation was that I would take a kit off her hands. Much as I love ferrets – I used to have one when I was a young boy – a pet ferret would be totally incompatible with my rabbits, so I had to decline. The best I could do was make a couple of phone calls and before long, acting as go-between, I'd managed to match up the last spare kit with a new owner.

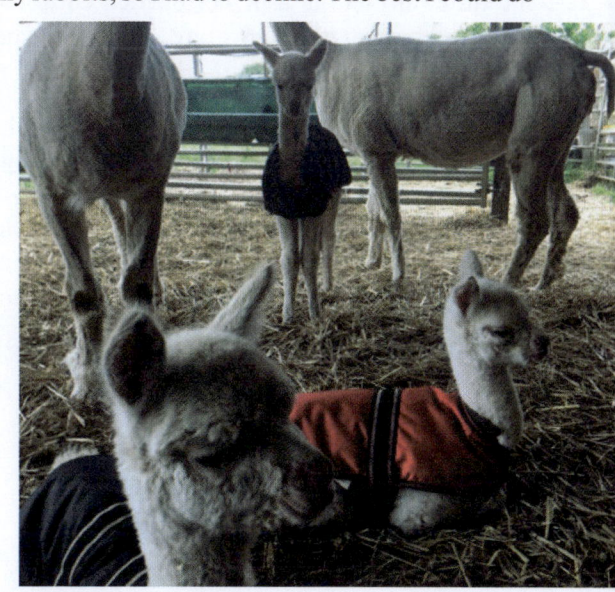

Later that week, I was surrounded by more babies. This time baby alpacas, which are called cria. Jackie had several newborns, and a visit for post-natal checks on both mothers and babies left me cooing with wonder at these amazing creatures. If you think a baby ferret is cute (which it is), then cria which are just a few days old take cuteness to a different level altogether. They look like balls of snow-white cotton wool on legs. Julia, a baby which I delivered a few weeks ago by emergency caesarean section, had not formed a proper bond with her mum. Or rather, her mum had not formed a proper bond with her, which is not uncommon after a caesarean because the natural hormones are not secreted sufficiently to trigger maternal bonds. This can be a problem, but not in Julia's case, because she quickly imprinted on Jackie herself and followed her around everywhere she went, much like Mary's little lamb.

As if that wasn't enough cute baby animals for one week, I was surprised to find a four-day-old chick waiting for me in afternoon surgery. It chirped and cheeped as it hopped around the basket in which it was transported. Apparently, its condition was called "pasty bottom", because it had, well, a pasty bottom. The little bird did not seem poorly, but the anxiety of the owner necessitated that I try to get to the bottom of the cause of the pasty bottom. As my swab went in to test for the pathogens which might be to blame, the little bird let out a higher pitched chirp than before, more by surprise than anything. We are all waiting patiently for the lab results, which should identify the cause.

Also waiting patiently was another ferret. Not a kit but an adult. He was waiting to get his pet passport so he could go on his holidays to Europe. The Pet Passport Scheme allows international travel between participating countries. It's applicable to dogs, cats and ferrets. I've never completed one for a ferret and nor has any vet I know, but everyone wants to. There is sure to be a big queue for this job too . . .

Goat with a Hairdo

I've seen quite a few goats recently. One of them belonged to Ian. He ran a mobile farm, the purpose of which was to visit schools, taking a multitude of animals to help educate young children. The goat was called "Starburst" and it had a swelling on its lower jaw. Ian was worried because the swelling had reached the size of a golf ball. On a pigmy goat, this was approximately the equivalent to a football-sized lump on a person. I headed down the A1 to investigate, armed with a sharp needle, a scalpel and plenty of excitement.

But it wasn't just Ian's goat that had a problem. His new business was foundering. Coronavirus restrictions meant that his trailer-load of interesting animals was housebound or, more accurately, farm-bound and the teaching, informing and enthusing of kids had ground to a halt. The country's recent and protracted lockdown was on the verge of claiming another victim. But, at least Starburst's facial problem could be treated without frightening any children.

Ian's farm was amazing. Animals of all shapes and sizes emerged from the far corners of fields and pens as I drove into the yard. Runner ducks appeared first. Upright and lengthy and rubbish at flying but, as their names suggested, adept at running. With their chests pushed up and out, they looked like sprinters approaching the finishing line, but waddling like a duck rather than loping gracefully like Usain Bolt. Ian explained how they were used in China to keep pests off rice plantations and in the vineyards of Italy to gobble up slugs. Apparently, they were more useful than their ridiculous appearance suggested. Next, there was a Polish chicken and a huge black turkey, which was doing her own gobbling, although not of slugs, as her baggy face wobbled side to side.

Attention turned to the patient, Starburst. The lump was prominent, but I was confident of an easy fix. Catching the frisky goat was the hardest part. As predicted, a sharp scalpel and a firm squeeze gave immediate relief to goat and satisfaction to the farmer and vet.

Another goat presented himself later in the week. Elvis had a spectacular but unwanted pair of testicles. He also had an amazing hairdo, which was just like the flamboyant hair of Lord Flashheart from *Blackadder*. Curled and quiffed, Elvis's locks were as impressive as the large testicles at the other end of his body – the area I'd be operating on. Goats are unusual in their intolerance of local anaesthetic. Even a small dose of this useful, and usually benign, drug can cause instant death. So, unlike in their ovine or bovine cousins, surgical procedures such as castration or jobs like removing the horn buds have to be done under full general anaesthetic. This was why Elvis had visited the practice today. The procedure was more similar to the castration of a dog than that of a calf. I held my breath as I injected the drugs to send Elvis to sleep. Administering unusual anaesthetics to irregular species can be a risky business, but fortunately Elvis's anaesthetic was smooth and uneventful, as was the removal of the mango-sized gonads. Elvis came around quickly and comfortably from the op to rid him of his manhood. Nurses and vets appeared to admire the handsome goat and his huge testicles, which now resided in a metal kidney dish rather than in their previous home of a caprine scrotum.

"Wow, what handsome . . ." exclaimed assorted staff. There were various words that followed that bit of the sentence. But, the op on the handsome goat with handsome testicles was finished and before long, without a care in the world, Elvis had left the building.

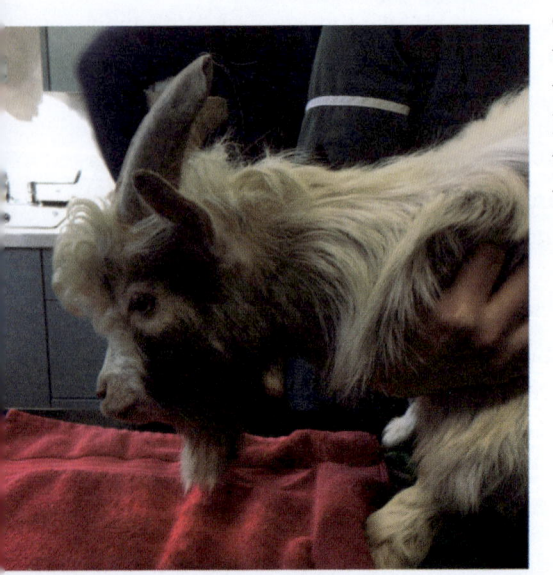

Vasectomising a Tup

The stocky texel tup, with eyes bulging from his bony head, looked like a battle-scarred rugby player. He had no idea what was in store for him. If he was able to string coherent thoughts together, he must have been confused that he'd been kept inside in an indoor pen on a pleasant summer's day. If he had known his fate, he certainly wouldn't have escaped through the chink in the door as I returned to my car to collect the important surgical equipment I needed.

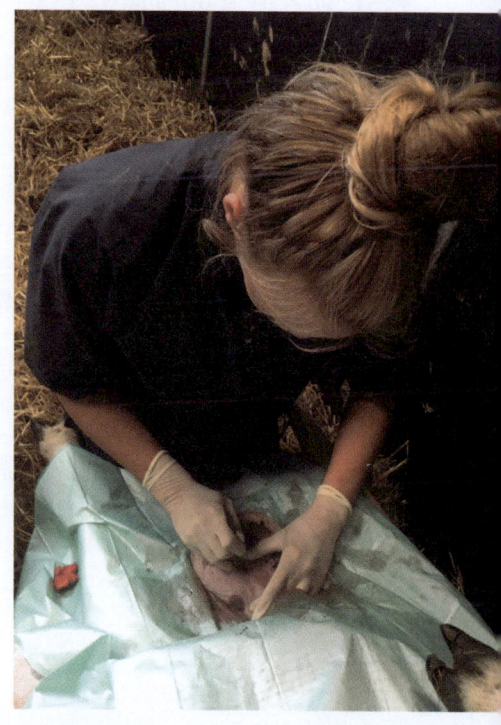

He was stronger than me, with a lower centre of gravity and powered by four legs rather than two, so I stood no chance of stopping him and my heart sank as he rushed past me in a blur and down the farm lane. It brought back bad memories of my first veterinary job when, as a newly qualified vet, I worked in Caithness at the very north of Scotland, in the practice now on its way to fame as *The Highland Vet*. A trailer appeared in the car park with two sheep, both suffering from vaginal prolapses. Since it was coffee time – a fiercely protected break in what were always very busy days – all the more senior vets had settled down to rest their weary legs. As a non-weary new graduate, overflowing with energy and enthusiasm, I jumped up to tackle the job, which should have been simple. Had both sheep not burst out over the tailgate and disappeared into the distance, it would have been simple. It *was* simple, once the furious, red-faced farmer and I had chased them down a lane for over a mile, before capturing them in a ditch.

Fortunately, there was no such similar drama today and the patient was quickly captured, using a bucket of tasty sheep nuts. Back in the stable, I arranged my equipment and awaited my colleague. The tup needed to be vasectomised. This is an excellent way to improve the efficiency of lambing time, by encouraging all the females to come into heat at the same time. For the male, it ensures a happy – a very happy – long life on the farm, mating to one's heart's content without fear of paternity issues, or the market.

Katy was coming to help/learn. At this stage of my veterinary career, I've lost count of the rams that I've vasectomised. Katy is still at the stage of being able to keep an accurate tally so, accomplished and adept as she already was, a chance for extra practice was grabbed with both hands. There is always something new to learn, even when you have been doing it for years. I did the first side, carefully cutting the pre-scrotal skin, identifying, transecting and then removing the all-important vas deferens. It was soon Katy's turn and we swapped positions between the ram's legs. It was hot, especially inside plastic trousers, a plastic top and latex gloves. With sweat dripping from my forehead and trickling down my back, I was happy to disrobe and defer the second part of the job.

"You should do it like this," Katy suggested, showing me a nifty technique to allow the patient's legs to be restrained with greater ease. A lambing rope looped over each hind foot and then knelt on by the surgeon provided a perfect way of keeping his legs out of the operating site. I have to say the second part of the surgery went more smoothly than the first. I could explain this by the fact that the right vas deferens rolls under the fingers more easily than the left, making its exposure easier. The truth is, of course, that Katy's surgical skills were already more honed and precise and her sutures more skilfully placed than mine. But it had been a useful afternoon. At least I'd learnt a new trick or two.

The Effects of Telly

Outside the practice, on a sunny day recently, I was accosted by several clients. I've been spending a lot of time standing outside the practice recently, mainly because of pesky COVID-19. Throughout the crisis, veterinary practices have been seeing patients, but have mitigated the risk of their staff being exposed to coronavirus by keeping owners outside. I know one practice that has erected a huge marquee, just like at a wedding, but rather than collecting a celebratory glass of fizz, pet owners and farmers stand two metres apart to hand over cat baskets or collect medicines. In the absence of a marquee in Boroughbridge, I've taken to speaking to clients on the pavement. There are downsides to this. One is that it is difficult when it rains or when the road-sweeper cleans the street; another is that passers-by stop and say hello, sometimes joining in the discussion. This happened recently.

"I'd like you to sign a card for my friend," explained an elderly Welsh lady, adding, "I'm not mad." I didn't think she was mad, because this sort of thing happens reasonably frequently to me. Being approached by strangers who think they know me personally is my new normal. But the elderly Welsh lady ("I'm from Wales, you know, but I live in York.") was obviously worried I would think she *was* mad and produced documentation from her cavernous bag, which she hoped would provide proof.

"I've brought my passport. Look, this is me," she offered, before following with more evidence of her identity. "And my driving licence."

This sort of documentation would suffice to apply for a mortgage. I thanked her, but reassured her that this was not necessary and that I did not think she was mad, nor did I need documentation to confirm her identity. Of course, this has all come about because of my appearance on *The Yorkshire Vet*, so I suppose, unintentionally, I've brought it upon myself. I don't mind. It's nice to be able to sign a birthday card for a sixty-seven-year-old lady who lives alone, because something as simple as writing in a card might bring some pleasure. I signed the card and she rummaged in her bag again.

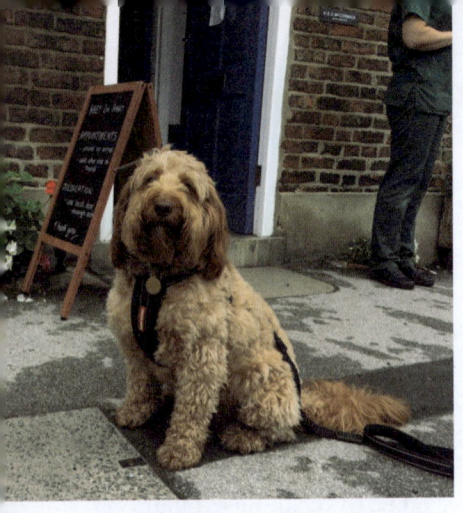

"This is a present to say thank you," she said, handing over four bottles of cider. "I found them in the garage."

On another day recently, again whilst standing on the practice doorstep waiting for a client, a second elderly lady, this time with a Jack Russell, went shuffling past. She chuckled, before explaining herself by saying simply, "You and that pig. My husband and I watch it endlessly. We can't stop laughing."

The endorsement, however, which rang most loudly, came from a lady who had made a special trip to see me from South Yorkshire. She was also clutching a bag, this time full of paperbacks. She asked if I could sign them.

"I've wanted to meet you and ask you to sign these books of yours," she explained. "It would mean a lot to me. My husband read them and then, as he became more poorly, I sat by his hospital bed and read them aloud. He loved your stories and I've wanted to come and let you know. You made a dying man very, very happy."

Once upon a time, I was just a vet and the fixing of an animal was the high point of the afternoon. Now, I've come to realise that other, less tangible things matter too. A book, which brings someone pleasure, or a comic moment in a TV series that makes someone laugh, can have just as profound an effect as curing a beloved cat.

Kirby Wiske

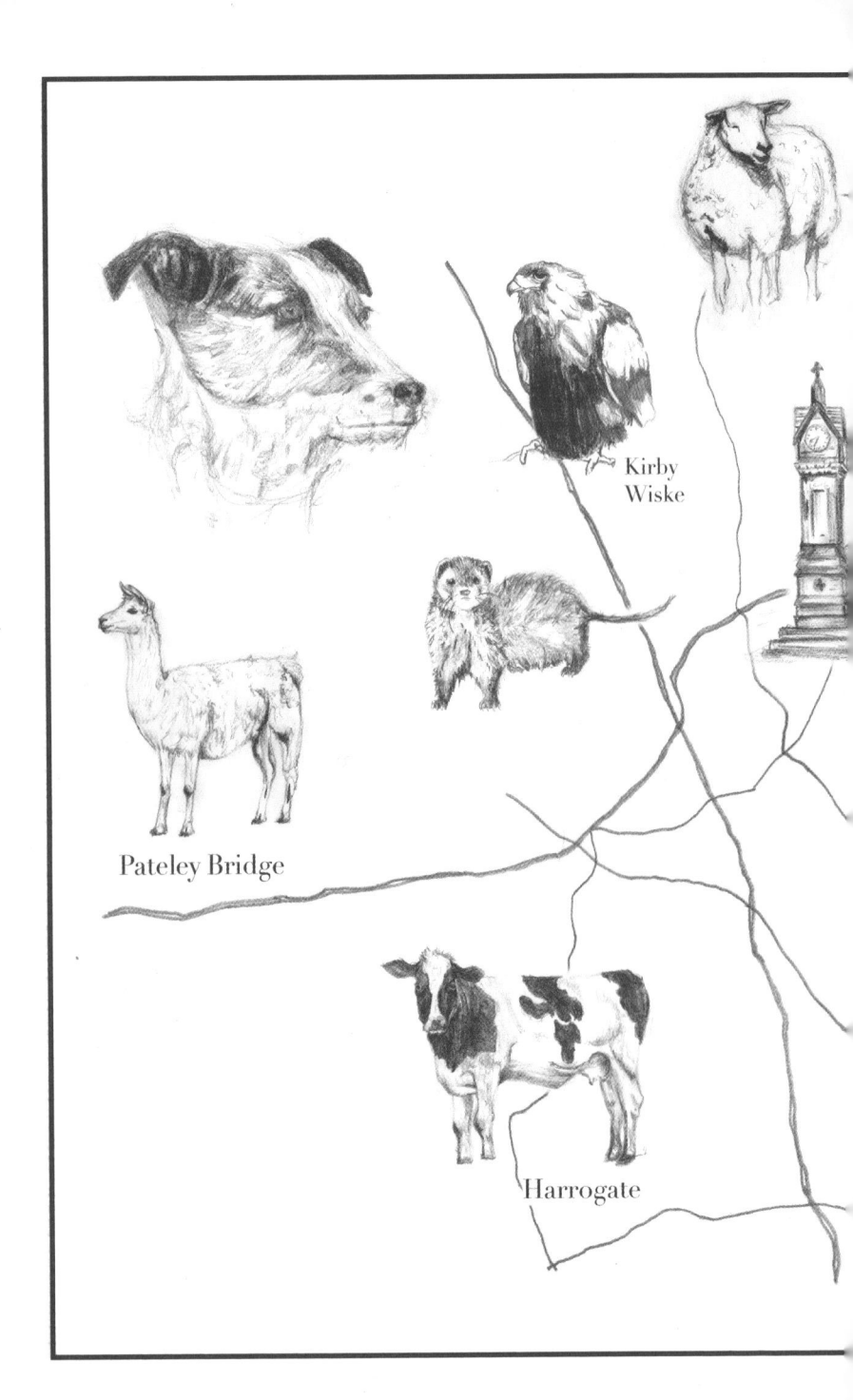

Pateley Bridge

Harrogate